WITHDRAWAL

VGM Opportunities Series

OPPORTUNITIES IN
BEAUTY CULTURE
CAREERS

Susan Wood Gearhart

Foreword by
Carol Cataldo
Executive Director
National Accrediting Commission of Cosmetology Arts
and Sciences

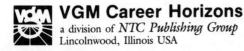 **VGM Career Horizons**
a division of *NTC Publishing Group*
Lincolnwood, Illinois USA

Cover Photo Credits:
Front cover: upper left, lower left, and lower
right, photos courtesy of Glemby; upper right,
Pittsburgh Beauty Academy.

Back cover: upper left, Chicago Cosmetologists
Association photo; upper right, photo courtesy
of Glemby; lower left, Pittsburgh Beauty
Academy photo; lower right, Helene Curtis
photo.

Library of Congress Cataloging-in-Publication Data

Gearhart, Susan Wood.
  Opportunities in beauty culture careers.

  (VGM opportunities series)
  Bibliography: p.
  Summary: Provides information on careers in beauty
culture including an overview of the field, educational
requirements, and employment outlook.
  1. Beauty culture—Vocational guidance. [1. Beauty
culture—Vocational guidance.   2. Vocational guidance]
  I. Title.   II. Series.
  TT958.G363   1988   646.7 '26 '02373   88-60910
  ISBN 0-8442-6518-7
  ISBN 0-8442-6519-5 (pbk.)

Published by VGM Career Horizons, a division of NTC Publishing Group.
© 1989 by NTC Publishing Group, 4255 West Touhy Avenue,
Lincolnwood (Chicago), Illinois 60646-1975 U.S.A.
Library of Congress Catalog Card Number: 88-60910
Manufactured in the United States of America.

8 9 0 BC 9 8 7 6 5 4 3 2 1

ABOUT THE AUTHOR

Susan Wood Gearhart is a professional model, dancer, teacher, free-lance writer, and editor. She graduated from City University of New York and attended Hiram College, Juilliard School, and the Preibar Academy in Berlin. She has modeled for several years for clothing, makeup, and hairstyles. She has developed programs for individual client skin care, skin sensitivity testing, and color coordination.

She has modeled for the major cosmetic firms of Estée Lauder, Clinique, Revlon, Charlie, Shiseido, and Ultima II, and has been a beauty and makeup design consultant for Clinique and Shiseido.

Ms. Gearhart lives in New York City.

ACKNOWLEDGMENTS

My gratitude and appreciation are extended to the following people for their kindness, help, and time. Among those to whom I want to express special thanks are: Daniel Kelley and Ms. Secas of Christine Valmy, New York City; Leo Galletta of the Atlas School of Barbering, New York City; Kathleen Paar of Clairol, NYC; Audrey Koppel of Kree Institute of Electrolysis, New York City; Ms. A. Ronni Kolotkin, Certified Electrologist; Mrs. Edith Imre and Mr. Michael of House Of Imre, New York City; Ms. Lurlie Calvacca, competition hairstylist and judge for competitions; Carlos Noceda, New York City; Nancy Tynan, Cosmair, Inc., L'Oréal International Salon Institute, New York City; Florence Lacoff, Cosmetological Publishing House, New York City; and Barbara W. Donner, former editor, National Textbook Company, Lincolnwood, Illinois.

FOREWORD

There are presently more than 1.7 million licensed cosmetologists in the United States and some 291,000 salons. Employment in the field of cosmetology is ample. Training in the field of cosmetology arts and sciences and related fields can prepare you for employment in a number of jobs, including hairstylist, salon manager, cosmetology teacher, manicurist, cosmetician, esthetician, platform artist, electrologist, and many more.

A career in cosmetology is one of great creativity and glamour. It is a profession that requires constant contact with people, one in which hard work and determination can result in rapid advancement. The first step toward a career in cosmetology is to pursue studies at a cosmetology school. By selecting one of the two thousand institutions accredited by the National Accrediting Commission of Cosmetology Arts and Sciences (NACCAS), you can be assured that the school meets certain educational standards.

Cosmetology schools are also regulated by state boards, which establish the length of the course, usually measured in hours, as well as course content. The length of the course varies, but for a basic cosmetology course you should anticipate devoting from six to ten months. Subsequently you must pass a state license exam to be able to practice.

The field of cosmetology is one of great variety. In addition to offering basic cosmetology courses, cosmetology schools may offer training in manicuring, salon management, and teacher training, as well as related specialties such as esthetics (skin care) and hair removal, both temporary and permanent.

With the aging of the baby boomers, there is a growing demand to look and feel good, which creates a demand for services in the beauty field. A world of beauty awaits those who wish to display their talent and creativity.

Carol Cataldo
Executive Director
National Accrediting Commission
of Cosmetology Arts and Sciences

PREFACE

Image-maker nonpareil! That could be your position as an operator in the beauty culture world. It's an exciting field as the masses gravitate toward popular television and movie stars for their hair and makeup idols and then to their hairstylists and makeup artists, who help them achieve similar looks. Makeup artists are next in demand behind hairstylists to keep the public not only well groomed but in the height of fashion. Millions of dollars are being spent, and that means thousands of positions are available in the cosmetology area to keep up with the need. Men and women are taking advantage of services today that only a handful of the population used just a few years ago.

As a hairstylist, manicurist, makeup artist, or hair colorist you will have the opportunity to help men and women come a little closer to their dreams of beauty. While you may not be able to make them as beautiful as the latest movie star, you can improve their appearance and help to give them a better image of themselves. And you can experience the personal satisfaction of making these people feel good about themselves. Last, but not least, you will earn the added reward of a good salary for your work.

The field of beauty culture is filled with opportunities. There are literally thousands of positions available. Your career could be as limited as a part-time shampooist in your local shopping mall, or you might become a famous hairstylist renowned for doing the hair of celebrities. Your personal ambitions will guide you to the best career for you.

I hope that this book will help you become aware of some of the many possibilities open to you. You will find that there is always a demand for talented beauticians. This demand helps to ensure that jobs will be both secure and rewarding. And since there are no employment limits because of sex or age, the beauty field offers a good future to any person who wants to pursue it.

With a few exceptions, state laws and codes that regulate the beauty field pertain to one state only. Health regulations and licensing vary greatly, as do age limits and pay scales. It is impossible to cover every detail in this general overview. Check with your state licensing agency. It will be extremely helpful in providing you with detailed information for your particular state.

If you are planning for a career in another state, be sure to write to that state's licensing agency well in advance of your move and in advance of your course plans. You will want to be completely familiar with the requirements and laws in the state where you will be working so that you can prepare accordingly.

INTRODUCTION

There are so many places of employment for a skilled professional in the beauty industry that it has become a sought-after field because of the financial security it offers. The need for cosmetologists in our country has stayed at the same number statistically for the past ten years. Trained professionals have come and gone at nearly the same rate because often the very young women who enter the field drop out and return in a few years after they have begun their families. The availability for work is generally good in all areas of our country.

The variety of specialized beauty services, the advancement of techniques, and the development of numerous hair, skin, and nail products have all had their impact upon the expansion of this labor market. There is simply a greater variety of cosmetologist posts as each area becomes highly specialized. Two areas that have experienced radical development are the hairstylist's and the manicurist's. Both have become so much in demand as creators of fashion and chic that there is often a problem trying to fit all the clients in!

Salaries for working cosmetologists vary radically in this industry because wages are based on the location of the salon, their level of experience, their following, and, of course, how they are actually paid. If their salary is based totally on percentage, commission, partial salary, and/or combinations of these financial arrangements, their salary will rise as the salon charges higher rates for its services. Not only does the economy set the standard for these increases, but the demand for fine work has a general effect on the prices that a place of work can charge. The more highly skilled technician has a tremendous advantage over the operator who has merely graduated from cosmetology school and has never kept up with continuing education in the field. Those who choose to apprentice after completing their state boards often find that they eventually earn a salary many times larger than their salaries would have been without the advanced training. Most people are more sophisticated now in their demands for a particular finished hairstyle or makeup, and this puts the burden of knowing how to accomplish that effect on the cosmetologist or cosmetician.

Cosmetology is a field that is as wide open to women as it is to men. The opportunities and potential for advancement are fairly distributed so that your ability and capability will dictate your success. This is a field where you must be self-motivated. There is no one who will push you, so if you desire to have a part-time job for only a few hours a week, you probably will be able to maintain that arrangement indefinitely. However, if your desire is to build a real career and to meet high goals, this is a perfect field for you to enter, as it offers you a limitless opportunity in your potential for growth.

Both men and women who choose to make cosmetology their chosen career will find it extremely rewarding. It does not have to be a full-time, six-day-a-week, all-out, all-consuming career. You can have a satisfying career in beauty culture even if you work only a few hours a week out of your own home. Nevertheless, the beauty field is an area where you can have a secure future with some of the best salaries in our country today being paid to women. The industry of cosmetology and its myriad jobs are extremely well paid. The jobs are many and challenging, and there is room to move around within certain spheres.

The current shift in employment is toward those with an indispensable technical skill and away from the college graduates. There are new beauty salons opening with regularity, and many positions are available in each one. The statistics show that more cosmetologists are self-employed (own their own salon) than other service workers. The overall outlook for cosmetology as a career is certainly an optimistic one. It is, however, a career where self-motivation is essential. But even for those people who are not interested in owning their own salons, cosmetology offers many opportunities. If you wish to work as a manicurist or hairdresser without the pressure to move upward, cosmetology can still be rewarding. The job is a pleasant one, and the relationship with the patrons can be very satisfying. Any service position is enjoyable if you genuinely like to please people and care about them.

DEDICATION

To Marguerite S. and Wm. Barker Wood,
Gabrielle, Jennifer and Ted

CONTENTS

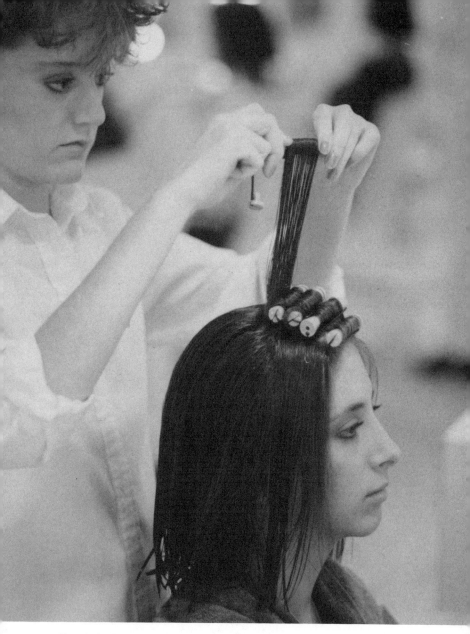

Cosmetologists work with their clients to help them improve their personal appearance. (Glemby International photo)

CHAPTER 1

BEAUTY CULTURE TODAY

A very few years ago, men and women went to the barber or beauty salon to look neater and to appear well-ordered. Today, most clients visit the hairstylist to maintain an image. Good grooming is very important to people, and they will pay great amounts of money to keep up the appearance of being blond, having hair, and generally having better looks than those nature endowed them with.

Hairstyles today are so complex that the client relies on the hairdresser for weekly maintenance as never before. The art of layering, perming, and coloring hair has become a much sought-after talent. There are hundreds of men and women who take advantage of all of these services. One very well-known colorist in New York City was so in demand by both sexes that he is now a salon owner and does coloring exclusively.

The expansion of the beauty field has made the techniques which were once available only to royal families and their courtiers accessible to everyone. For centuries, women longed to copy the makeup enhancing Cleopatra's eyes, the wigs adorning Marie Antoinette, and the long tapered fingernails of wealthy ladies. Today, the hairdresser is trained to give you an attractive style by knowing just what color, haircut, and proportion will look best for you. Through the perfection of chemical technology and the caliber of advanced teaching techniques, it is literally astounding how different cosmetology can make someone look.

There are endless combinations of haircuts, styles, and perms, and endless mixes of hair colors, including the really brilliant tones now popular. It is not unusual to see a dancer in a night spot with multi-colored hair, silver-streaked hair, or even period hairstyles from the past decades.

Hairstyles vary widely according to where you live, your age group, and, of course, the occasion. Evening, for example, may call for more elaborate makeup than school or work. The face must be made to look its best for every occasion, be it the daily job or the special night out.

Every one of us has an image of him or herself. Regardless of how attractive others may view you, if you are unhappy with your own image, you are uneasy. The choice to be as you see yourself is what cosmetology is all about. Many beauty techniques merely fool the eye by taking into consideration facial shapes and altering appearances to draw attention to good features or away from bad ones. Color also will make the viewer see features differently. Lighter hair dyes can make some patrons look very beautiful while others look very "washed out"; darker colors may look too heavy on one and rich and dramatic on another.

COMMON BEAUTY TREATMENTS

Electrolysis

Electrolysis is a technique that removes unwanted hair from all parts of the body. Most often it is facial hair that is removed by this process. Suppose that you have very thick, dark eyebrows. Although you have plucked them repeatedly, your eyebrows are still too heavy to allow your eyes to be seen to their best advantage. Electrolysis could permanently tweeze those thick brows away. Your face will look different every time you alter one of your characteristics. It is as wonderful and exciting to see these transformations as it is to see the pleasure that they instill.

Manicures

Fingernails and hands are also important to one's self-image. Long tapered nails disguise short fingers and emphasize long fingers. Nail polish also draws attention to hands and can be used as a fashion accessory to any costume. If you are not lucky enough to have lovely nails of your own, there are several methods of creating those even, long, or special shapes that you might desire. The technique of strengthening nails can sometimes alleviate problems due to chipping, cracking, or splitting. If the nails are so weak that physical correction is impossible, the tips can be built up with artificial materials, or a whole plastic nail can be attached over the natural nail. There has always been a fascination with women having long fingernails, but it is very important to have well-groomed hands and nails, regardless of the nails' length. Men and women alike need to present themselves with attractive nails, so the manicurist has an important job.

Cutting Hair

Hair length, like many other apsects of beauty, is partially dictated by fashion. Sometimes long hair is in vogue; at other times it seems that all the fashion models have short hair. Hair length can also be influenced by your personal preferences and individual features. If you have too little hair for current trend, you might incorporate a fall or hairpiece. Too much hair could make you consider a thinning with special shears. An altogether inappropriate hair color, texture, amount, length, or cut could send you looking for a good wig.

Skin Care

Facial problems also produce many jobs in the beauty field. *Skin care specialists* carefully analyze the problems of too much or too little natural oil in the skin and prescribe corrective measures. Massages are also a part of the skin care specialist's routine. Heat, cold, electrical stimulation, creams, and facial packs are all employed in the skin's care.

Makeup

Makeup is a rapidly expanding field of its own. There are many job opportunities for the person who specializes in makeup. There is such a demand for demonstration of beauty products in some of the larger cities that agencies have formed to handle makeup artists exclusively. The positions can be anything from applying makeup to a television actress before a show or commercial to doing a make over on an airline stewardess in her training school program. The hair and makeup of famous movie stars are creations of these cosmetologists.

Special effects are as sought after in makeup as in any of the other fashion markets. As a makeup artist you could specialize in corrective makeup to conceal birthmarks, scars, or irregular pigmentation. A clever makeup artist is highly sought after and highly paid.

RESEARCH

Laboratories provide challenging jobs for those interested in the chemical end of cosmetology. Products need to be formulated correctly so that people who use the cosmetics will benefit and not have an allergic reaction. Both the creation of new products and the improvement of standard products are the work of *chemists.* A college degree is required for this job.

The person who tests the formulas on the customer is a *product formulation tester.* His or her work consists of experimenting with the actual new product on the patron's hair or skin. These patrons do not pay for the work done since they are taking a small risk that they may not react well to the new product. But they usually receive very good hair and facial care because the licensed cosmetologist who does the testing has had the benefit of many years of experience before being advanced to the position of formulation tester.

MANAGEMENT AND TEACHING

Career possibilities also lie in owning, managing, or instructing at a beauty school or salon. As long as you have the capital to invest, you can be a partner or an owner of a beauty salon or beauty school. There are laws in the various states that govern the amount of space required for a salon or school, and the size needed certainly affects the investment required.

Depending on the size of the school or salon, one person might both own and manage the business as well as work on hair. In larger salons where there are many employees, the manager sees to hiring, time schedules, and appointments. He or she sets up demonstrations and coordinates the entire working machinery of the salon. Obviously a large salon with many patrons would bring larger responsibility and a higher salary.

The position of instructor not only requires that you be licensed by the state, but also that you have completed education courses offered by a college or university. The length of study for the required college credits varies from state to state. The position also requires extensive patience, as do all teaching posts. Teaching is a separate field. You could be the best hairdresser in the country and not qualify as an instructor. Many fine hairstylists give up in anger, cut the patron's hair, and leave a bewildered student wondering how to give that particular haircut. No matter how slowly a student learns, an instructor must go over techniques again and again until the procedure is fully understood.

I have spoken with really superb hairstylists who admit not passing their state exams the first time around, who determinedly went back to school until they understood the techniques. For some the process was quite extended, but their ambition and determination has put them in demand of patrons who are willing to pay highly for excellence.

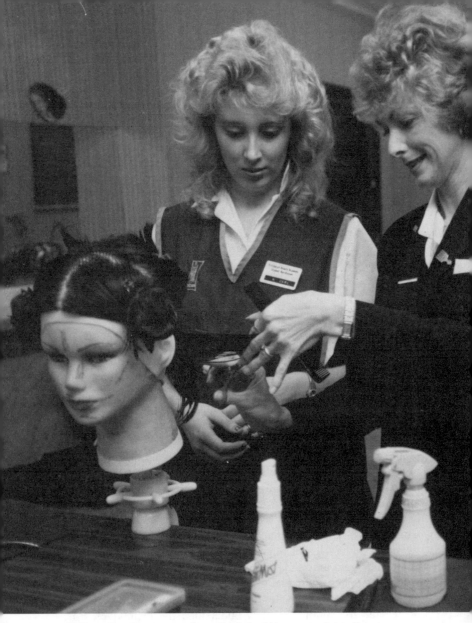

Students choosing a cosmetology school should be aware of state licensing requirements and the quality of the school's curriculum and instructors. (Pittsburgh Beauty Academy photo)

CHAPTER 2

CHOOSING A SCHOOL AND OBTAINING A LICENSE

SCHOOLS

Unfortunately for the cosmetology licensee, regulations are determined by each individual state. You may be living in one state and desire to relocate to another. You probably will have to be relicensed, which could entail extra schooling or, at least, lost time and wages while you are fulfilling your new license requirements. Laws have been proposed to alleviate this problem and to federalize cosmetology standards so that one license would permit you to work in all fifty states.

Read carefully all the regulations that pertain to your state's licensing and write to your state's department of education to clarify as much as possible the hours required and reciprocal understandings with any other states. You don't want to find yourself holding a license for a state that falls short in hours and credits if you know that you don't intend to stay there.

It would be impossible to list every beauty school or to point out every advantage of getting your cosmetology education at one school or another. But we will try to cover several types of cosmetology educational offerings located in several states to give you an idea of what is generally available.

Public Schools

Schools offering beauty courses break down into three categories. The first of this group is the public school. Many schools offer cosmetology courses at an introductory level. In Florida, for example, high school students can enroll in cosmetology instruction in high schools, in area vocational-technical centers, and in community colleges.

Selecting an approved public cosmetology school can save you time and money. If you take cosmetology courses at a public school during your high school years, you can avoid the usual beauty school fees. In many high schools, students enter a beauty program in the eleventh grade for three hours every day. In the summer, they take training for six hours a day, and they take three hours a day of courses during the twelfth grade. In the vocational centers and community colleges, classroom time varies. If a student has completed all required subjects, he or she will attend classes for five to six hours a day. All postsecondary training is taught at a rate of five to six hours each day with the entire courses taking anywhere from 600 to 1,200 hours, as required by law. The individual school must certify that the student is ready for the state board examination.

Some states, such as Florida, have an extensive system of public cosmetology schools located in high schools, education centers, vocational centers, junior colleges, community colleges, adult programs, and adult centers. These technical facilities are scattered all over the state so they can be easily reached. Even the Florida School for the Deaf and Blind at St. Augustine offers cosmetology as a career.

There are eighty approved public cosmetology schools in Florida, if both day and evening schools are taken into consideration. Two of these are housed within correctional institutions.

California has many public schools where cosmetology is offered. A list of these qualified establishments may be obtained by writing to the California State Board of Cosmetology, in care of the California Department of Consumer Affairs. Part-time attendance at a school of cosmetology will meet California law requirements that everyone must attend public school until their eighteenth birthday. After a person reaches that age, he or she can take cosmetology courses full time, and then be licensed. California has no continuing education requirements.

California's public cosmetology programs are in colleges, vocational centers, high schools, junior colleges, occupational centers, and adult schools. There are thirty-one schools listed in the state's catalog.

Several other states also offer comprehensive cosmetology programs in their public school system. The junior year in high school seems the normal time to start these classes. If you are interested in taking cosmetology courses while you are still in high school, and your school does not offer any program, check with your local school administration for any possible classes in the area. Try to locate a school where you can take advantage of cosmetology instruction.

There are some schools that are neither strictly public nor private. You will pay a small amount of money for your education, but because of state funds within that particular school, your tuition will be much less than a private beauty school. These are considerations that you will want to take into account before you decide upon a school.

Private Schools

The second category of cosmetology schools is the private school. There are extensive differences in some of the schools due to instructors, standards of education required of the instructor, and the attitude and ability of the manager of the school. One very clever young lady revealed her technique for the best way to find the right school: Go to the best salons in town and ask their newest operators and apprentices where they took basic training. One way of judging the quality of a school's curriculum is to find out whether or not a school's graduates are getting jobs after graduation. After all, that is your primary concern.

You may already know that a particular salon is your choice for work, so don't be shy about talking to its manager and finding out his or her preferences in cosmetology graduates. He or she will be glad to tell you. The manager is running a successful business and intends to keep up its standards by hiring well-instructed graduates.

Choosing a School

There are probably many beauty schools in your community, so make a list of all the ones that you might consider and call for an appointment. Try to sit in on a full day of work, instruction, and practice classes. If your area does not have a school that will let you sit in on classes, at least try to meet the classroom instructor and manager of the school. You will get a better idea of how the institution is run if you have the chance to communicate with the administrator directly. Remember that you are going to be paying to learn. By learning as much as you can about a school before you pay your tuition, you can help to guarantee that you will receive a good education. Fees vary widely depending on your locale, but you can expect to pay anywhere from $1,800 upward for the minimum hours of schooling. In New York City, it would not be unusual to pay over $3,000 for the school's required hours. But even with the best school, there is no guarantee that you will graduate. If you do not pass your state exams, you may have to return for more schooling at your own expense. So make a careful choice. Once you have committed yourself to the idea of becoming a cosmetologist, work hard and don't be discouraged if things seem to move at a snail's pace. Nothing is easy at the beginning, and every cosmetologist that I have spoken with admits that beauty school, like all schools, is a challenge. You will experience satisfaction and a feeling of accomplishment for many years after you have mastered your craft.

The years needed to complete your cosmetology schooling will vary according to how much time you are able to give your classes and practical assignments. If you attend full time, you could finish your schooling in as little as eight months. "Full time" would mean an eight-hour day, holidays excluded. If you attend only in the evenings, you would take about twice as long to complete the required hours. Of course, every state is different, and some require as many as 2,000 school hours, so you would finish in a little longer period of time. You might be going to classes as much as eight hours a day or as little as a few hours on Saturdays only. The less concentrated the time, the longer the course. Another curious thing that appears in some manuals is that a beauty school hour is only fifty-five minutes long. Be sure to ask about it so that both you and your faculty come out with the same total at the end.

Schools Offering Advanced Training

The last category of schools is the group that offers advanced training in cosmetology. This group is mentioned only briefly, as you may or may not elect to attend advanced training. In certain beauty salons, new techniques are demonstrated by permanent or traveling instructors. These new methods are shown to operators so that they can incorporate the current styles or trends that have just come into fashion. Fashion is constantly changing, and makeup and hairstyles must keep up with the latest "look." If you are an operator whose patrons demand the latest haircuts and styles, and your salon does not provide a periodic demonstrator, you will want to attend master classes to learn some fine points. In these classes, you will benefit from the experience and wisdom of a well-established professional hairstylist. It may be someone who is well known as a competition hair designer, a precision cutter, or a recognized colorist. Any added knowledge that you acquire will surely mean added clients and, of course, the compensatory salary and tips. These special schools may appear to be extremely expensive, but the $100 or more you pay for the day's class could mean a large difference in your income.

Financial Aid

Financial aid is available in various states. As you might suspect, the aid is proportional to your own ability to pay. Aid can be obtained as a grant, which does not have to be repaid, or in the form of a loan that must be paid back. Most beauty schools have information about the types of financial assistance that you may be eligible for. Some of the financial aid programs for which you may qualify are Basic Educational Opportunity Grants (BEOG), Supplementary Educational Opportunity Grants (SEOG), National Direct Student Loans (NDSL), and Guaranteed Student Loans (GSL). When you consider any cosmetology schools, these are the programs that you will want to investigate if you need assistance. Remember that these programs, too, may change; but as new titles and programs become available, you will learn of them only by being constantly in touch, asking questions, and keeping informed. Ask for brochures on the available programs so that you will be able to think them through clearly before you make any agreements to take a loan. Not all schools that teach cosmetology are qualified to give financial help. There are government regulations that dictate policy on giving money for tuition.

There are also agencies in the larger cities that try to help you find financial aid after you are enrolled. If you find yourself unable to keep up your tuition payments, it would be foolish not to take a loan, especially if you find yourself near to completing the required hours. To start over again at a later date would probably be extremely costly. Tuitions are constantly rising in the private cosmetology catalogs. But it is of paramount importance that you complete the minimum schooling at one time. Otherwise the critical knowledge you need for your state boards may be too dated or drawn out for you to remember.

APPRENTICESHIPS

After you have completed your state licensing, you may want to apprentice in a better salon. The purpose behind this is to develop as a good hairstylist and earn an excellent salary. If you desire to be associated with a salon with a reputation for high style or trendsetting, you must be prepared to accept very low compensation while you closely observe a well-established operator in that particular salon. You will be expected to put in normal working hours (usually an eight-hour day), and do everything that is asked of you by the busy top hairstylists. This could include shampooing, assisting with hair treatments, holding hair clips, and drying hair. You will not do haircutting or final styling until you have learned all the fine points of the specialized techniques. You could apprentice for as many as five to seven years in a very elaborate salon. It all depends on your ability to learn to cut hair with dexterity and cleverness. There are specific haircuts and styles that better known salons have made famous. To learn a detailed type of cut is painstaking but absolutely necessary.

Apprentices Prior to Certification

Not all states have regulations that permit students to apprentice before securing a license. An apprentice is someone who learns by on-the-job training. The difference in this type of apprenticeship from the type just discussed is that this type of apprentice is clearly a trainee and has not yet accumulated the required educational hours to take the state boards. In some states where apprentices are schooled in beauty salons, state regulations will designate in every detail the registration requirements for the apprentice and the instructor-to-apprentice ratio in the place of business. In states that permit apprentices, strict laws stipulate all the conditions under which apprentices may be trained. These laws are clearly stated in the brochures put out by the specific state. If you are considering training as an apprentice prior to taking your state boards, it is imperative that you read all materials pertinent to registered apprentices. The fee paid by apprentices is not listed in most advertising brochures. Also, be sure to make inquiries at your local beauty salon to see where you actually would take all of the needed courses. They may or may not be given in the same location.

Apprenticeships also vary in actual required hours from state to state. The average appears to be two years of noncertified, but registered, apprenticeship in a beauty salon under the tutelage of the designated number of certified operators. The required years of work would differ according to the individual's capabilities.

LICENSING REQUIREMENTS

Minimum Age and Schooling

The minimum age and amount of formal schooling required for licensure differ from state to state. So before you make plans to enroll in any cosmetology course be sure to find out the minimum age at which you can get a license. Some states don't even permit the state examinations until a particular age, so determine when you will be able to take the exam before you enroll. The average age for entry into cosmetology schools seems to be sixteen. Average schooling requirements vary much more widely. In Texas, for example, you can enroll in cosmetology school at the age of fifteen, and you need only have completed the seventh grade in elementary school. In Washington, D.C., you need only to have completed the eighth grade, but must be sixteen years old. So you can see that there is a large variance in licensing requirements among the states.

Some states allow special testing for people who do not speak English well. If English is not your first language, investigate your state laws through a translator. Many states provide a practical test rather than a written test for those who do not speak English.

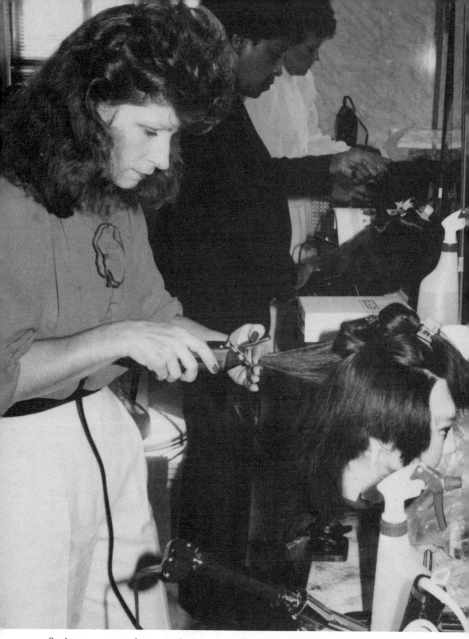

Students must complete a required number of school hours before they can apply to take state board examinations. (Chicago Cosmetological Association photo)

Application for Licensure

Once you have completed the required number of school hours for your state, you must apply to take the state board examinations. Your state has forms that are prescribed by the state cosmetology board. Every state has different time schedules to be followed, and you should check to see how far in advance you need to apply to take the exams at the designated time. You may find that application has to be made weeks or months in advance. So even if you have not yet graduated from beauty school, look into scheduling your exam.

There is also a fee, called the initial licensing fee, that must be paid to the state when you take your state boards. You will want to set that amount aside ahead of time.

When the time comes to actually obtain your license, inquire about renewal procedures. Your license is not a lifetime affair. It has to be renewed once every year in some states and once every two years in others. Most states have a set month wherein you are to renew cosmetology licenses. In New York, for instance, cosmetology licenses are renewed on July 1. Check with your state and any other where you may want to work in the future to learn about procedures. Because of large amounts of paperwork, state departments are always very slow, so licensing takes time. Be sure that you have proper licensing so that waiting to receive a license does not cost you working days.

Reciprocity between states means that if you are a licensed operator in one state, your training is recognized by many other states with similar cosmetology licensing rules and regulations. Wherever required hours and courses are alike, you probably will be able first to attain a temporary license from the new state, and then acquire a permanent license. Again, time will be of the essence. State departments are not intentionally trying to slow you down or prevent you from working, but you should allow several months in most states to receive all the necessary documents after you have made your initial application.

Licensing Examination

There is a National Cosmetology Examination now offered in thirty states. This test, consisting of one hundred questions, can be as long as one-and-a-half hours or as short as one hour. Records of the test are kept in the National Interstate Council of State Boards of Cosmetology.

There are special books now in print that will help you study either to pass the regular state boards in your state or the national examination. The books will help you to know what to expect in the exams and how to conduct yourself at the examination. They also give you sample questions to test your knowledge in all the areas that you are expected to understand. When you know what to expect and what types of questions will be asked, you will be much better prepared and less worried about either the written or the practical tests.

Ask at your local bookstore for the books; if they are not in stock, the bookstore can order them for you so you can brush up on all the work that you have covered in your cosmetology course.

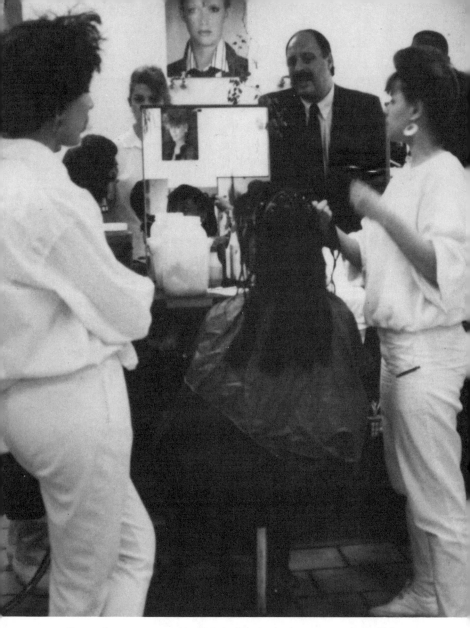

Cosmetology courses combine technical instruction by experts and practical operation with the student actually performing a service on another person or on a mannequin. (Capri School of Beauty Culture, Inc. photo)

CHAPTER 3

COSMETOLOGY STUDY

Basic cosmetology courses vary from state to state. State laws are very slow to change, and though many are being considered for revision, no new laws have been enacted that alter the curriculum examples that follow.

CURRICULUM

The curriculum for students enrolled in a cosmetologist course in California consists of 1,600 clock hours of technical instruction and practical operations. The courses cover all practices constituting the art of cosmetology.

For the purpose of this section, *technical instruction* means instruction by demonstration, lecture, classroom participation, or examination. *Practical operation* is defined as the actual performance by the student of a complete service on another person or on a mannequin. According to the State Board of Cosmetology, California Administrative Code, Ch. 9, Title 16, these include:

Subject	Minimum Hours of Technical Instruction	Minimum Practical Operation
1. *The Cosmetology Act and the Board's Rules and Regulations*	20	
2. *Cosmetology Chemistry*—the chemical composition and purpose of cosmetic, nail, hair, and skin preparations. Shall also include the elementary chemical makeup, physical, and chemical changes of matter.	20	
3. *Theory of Electricity in Cosmetology*—the nature of electric current, principles of operating electrical devices, and the various safety precautions used when operating electrical equipment.	5	
4. *Safety*—bacteriology, sterilization and sanitation, safety precautions, anatomy, and physiology.	30	
5. *Wet Hairstyling*—hair analysis, shampooing, fingerwaving, pin curling, and combouts.	25	250
6. *Thermal Hairstyling*—hair analysis, straightening, waving, curling with hot combs and hot curling irons, and blower styling.	15	45
7. *Permanent Waving*—hair analysis, chemical and heat permanent waving.	20	100
8. *Chemical Straightening*—hair analysis and the use of sodium hydroxide and other basic solutions.	15	15

Subject	Minimum Hours of Technical Instruction	Minimum Practical Operation
9. *Haircutting*—hair analysis and the use of razor, scissors, electric clippers, and thinning shears for wet and dry cutting.	25	100
10. *Haircoloring and Bleaching*—hair analysis, predisposition tests, safety precautions, formula mixing, tinting, bleaching, and the use of dye removers.	40	70
11. *Scalp and Hair Treatments*—hair and scalp analysis, scientific brushing, electric and manual scalp manipulation, and other hair treatments.	5	50
12. *Facials* A. Manual—cleansing, scientific manipulations, packs, and masks.	5	15
B. Electrical—the use of all electrical modalities, including dermal lights and electrical apparatus for facials and skin care purposes.	15	15
13. *Eyebrow Arching and Hair Removal*—the use of wax, electric or manual tweezers, and depilatories for the removal of superfluous hair.	5	15
14. *Makeup*—skin analysis, complete and corrective makeup, and the application of false eyelashes.	15	10

Subject	Minimum Hours of Technical Instruction	Minimum Practical Operation
15. *Manicuring and Peducuring—* A. Water and oil manicure—including nail analysis and hand and arm massage.	5	25
B. Complete pedicure—including nail analysis and foot and ankle massage.	2	5
C. Artificial Nails—including liquid and powder brush-ons, artificial nail tips, and nail wraps and repairs.	10	30
16. *Additional Training—*may include professional ethics, personal hygiene, good grooming, salesmanship, normal cleanup duties, keeping of student records, patron service record cards, modeling, desk and reception, and care and styling of wigs; may also include not more than sixteen hours' credit for field trips. Field trips must be under the direct supervision of a licensed cosmetology instructor.	100	
All students who have completed the specified minimum required hours have completed the educational requirements for licensure in California.		

A second example of a beauty school curriculum comes from a catalog advertisement. This particular cosmetology school is located in New York City. The classes represent what you could expect to learn there in eight months.

Course	Total Hours
1. Fingerwaving	200
2. Permanent Waving	175
3. Haircutting and Hairstyling	125
4. Dyes, Bleaches, and Rinses	100
5. Scalp Treatment	50
6. Shampoos	25
7. Manicuring	100
8. Facials	50
9. Sanitation, Sterilization, Hygiene, and Anatomy	50
10. Tests and Exams	25
11. Shop Management and Business Ethics	50
12. Nondesignated Time	50
Total	1,000

After the completion of the diversified courses in the cosmetology curriculum, you may find yourself doing any or all of the various jobs in a beauty salon. Or you may want to specialize.

SPECIALIZED COURSES

In many states, if you hold a specialty certificate, you are permitted to work in only one particular field. The following definitions of specialties were taken from the General Rules and Regulations including the Cosmetology Commission Sanitary Rulings from the Texas Cosmetology Commission.

Cosmetologist—A cosmetologist (operator) license authorizes the holder to practice all phases of cosmetology in a beauty salon or any specialties in a specialty shop.

Wig specialist—A wig specialist certificate authorizes the holder to practice wiggery, hairweaving, or perform eye tabbing in a beauty or specialty salon.

Manicurist—A person holding a manicurist license may perform for compensation only the practices of manicuring and pedicuring in a licensed beauty or specialty salon.

Shampoo conditioning specialist—A shampoo specialist certificate authorizes the holder to practice the art of shampooing, application of conditioners and rinses, scalp manipulation, and sell shampooing hair goods in a licensed beauty or specialty salon.

Facial specialist—A facial specialist certificate authorizes the holder to practice facials, application of facial cosmetics, manipulations, eye tabbing, arches, lash and brow tints, and the temporary removal of facial hair in a licensed beauty or specialty salon.

Hairweaving specialist—A hairweaving specialist certificate authorizes the holder to practice the art of hairweaving in a licensed beauty or specialty salon.

There are many areas in which you may desire to specialize. As you can see from the certifications, you might be able to go directly into a special field with only a set curriculum for your selected area. Or you may have to complete all the required hours in your state, take your state boards, and then specialize. In states with specialty certificates you cannot perform activities not designated by law. To do so might cause you to have your license revoked. Not all states allow specialty certification courses, but most states do have manicuring-only classes for certification.

LIMITED CERTIFICATES

In some states, you will discover that the license is called a limited certificate. A limited certificate is one that takes only a few school hours to complete. Anywhere between one hundred and three hundred hours could qualify you for a manicurist certificate, for example. A proportionate number of hours are designated to teach you all you need to know on that one topic.

Limited course offerings in cosmetology schools can qualify you to take the state boards in that one special field. Here is a school description of a manicurist course:

Course	Total Hours
1. Orientation	4
2. Manicure Tools and Use	9
3. Nail Structure (Theory)	1
4. Sterilization and Sanitation	2
5. Manicuring Procedure and Hand Massage	84
6. Manicuring Practices	7
7. Manicuring for Men	3
8. Tests	3
Total	150

Remember also that in some states, there is no license requirement for manicurists, wig stylists, receptionists in beauty schools, and assistant manager positions.

SUPPLEMENTAL COURSES

There are supplementary courses offered in some states to give a wider scope to your original learning. These extensions are aimed at helping you develop additional talents in your own field. Suppose that you had gone to barbering school, had become very much in demand, and were offered a position to dress the hair and do the makeup for a traveling rock group. Since you are only licensed to style hair, that would limit your work, and the rock group requires that only one cosmetician travel with them. What you could do is quickly return to school. But this time you would take your barber's certification to a beauty school and take a shortened course.

Not every state has this type of arrangement, but it is a great convenience if it exists. The following is an example of one program designed for barbers who want to get their cosmetology licenses. The curriculum, excerpted from the State of California Administrative Code, consists of four hundred clock hours of technical instruction and practical operations over the required training of a barber. For the purpose of this section, *technical instruction* means instruction by demonstration, lecture, classroom participation, or examination. *Practical operation* refers to the actual performance by a student of a complete service on another person or on a mannequin. Such instruction shall include:

Subject	Minimum Hours of Technical Instruction	Minimum Practical Operation
1. *The Cosmetology Act and the Board's Rules and Regulations*	10	
2. *Cosmetology Chemistry*—the chemical composition and purpose of cosmetic, nail, hair, and skin preparations. Shall also include the elementary chemical makeup, physical, and chemical changes of matter.	5	
3. *Theory of Electricity in Cosmetology*—the nature of electric devices, and the various safety precautions used when operating electrical equipment.	5	
4. *Safety*—bacteriology, sterilization and sanitation, safety precautions, anatomy, and physiology.	5	

Subject	Minimum Hours of Technical Instruction	Minimum Practical Operation
5. *Wet Hairstyling*—hair analysis, fingerwaving, pin curling, and combouts.	10	35
6. *Thermal Hairstyling*—hair analysis, straightening, waving, curling with hot combs and hot curling irons.	5	15
7. *Permanent Waving*—hair analysis, sectioning patterns, chemical and heat permanent waving.	10	35
8. *Chemical Straightening*—hair analysis and the use of sodium hydroxide and other base solutions.	5	10
9. *Haircutting*—hair analysis, basic guideline and sectioning, the use of the razor, scissors for wet and dry cutting.	2	10
10. *Haircoloring and Bleaching*—hair analysis, predisposition tests, safety precautions, formula mixing, tinting, bleaching, and the use of dye removers.	20	20
11. *Scalp and Hair Treatments*—hair analysis, scientific brushing.	2	5
12. *Facials* A. Manual—cleansing, scientific manipulations, packs, and masks.	2	5
B. Electrical—the use of all electrical modalities, including dermal lights and electrical apparatus for facials and skin care purposes.	10	10

Subject	Minimum Hours of Technical Instruction	Minimum Practical Operation
13. *Eyebrow Arching and Hair Removal*—the use of wax, electrical or manual tweezers, and depilatories for the removal of superfluous hair.	5	5
14. *Makeup*—skin analysis, complete and corrective makeup, and the application of false eyelashes.	5	10
15. *Manicuring and Pedicuring*— A. Water and oil manicure—nail analysis and hand and arm massage. B. Complete pedicure—nail analysis and foot and ankle massage. C. Artificial Nails—liquid and powder brush-ons, artificial nail tips, and nail wraps and repairs.	5 1 5	15 3 15
16. *Additional Training*—professional ethics, salesmanship, normal cleanup duties, required keeping of student records, patron service record cards, and modeling. The course may also include not more than eight hours credit for field trips. Field trips must be under the direct supervision of a licensed cosmetology instructor.	25	

TRAINING FOR INSTRUCTORS

Another whole area of specialization involves the instruction or teaching fields. There are many positions open to instructors, demonstrators, and even lecturers in the cosmetology field. Some states require special education courses for these posts while others demand only a license in cosmetology from that state and several years of experience as a practicing cosmetician. If you are interested in a teaching job, the best way to find out the details is to write your state's board of education and find out the current prerequisites. The department can also supply you with the list of all public and private schools of cosmetology where you will be qualified to instruct. Be sure to find out when your license expires and keep it up-to-date. You need to hold a cosmetology license to teach. If you find that your license has expired, you could waste a great deal of time getting it back again.

MANAGERIAL AND BUSINESS POSITIONS

Managerial posts may interest you. There are many of these jobs in department store beauty salons, specialty shops, beauty shops, facial schools, facial salons, cosmetology schools, electrology schools, wiggeries, and cosmetic businesses.

Last, but not least, your specialty may be in the business end of the cosmetology world. You may want to own a chain of shops or salons. Although this is not likely to be an immediate accomplishment, you may want to start with owning one beauty salon as soon as possible. It is really quite common to see several salons owned by the same proprietor. Some people have very good business minds. You could combine your talents as a cosmetician and your competitive abilities by owning your own beauty school or salon.

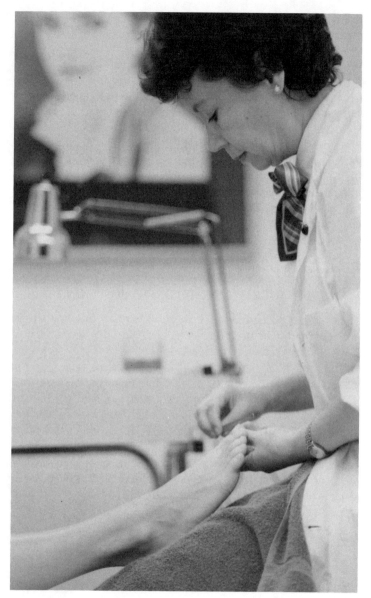

Nail care specialists work in beauty salons or in independent nail salons.
(Glemby International photo)

CHAPTER 4

THE NAIL SALON

MANICURISTS AND PEDICURISTS

Revolutionary strides have been taken in the nail care field. The specialty has so diversified that the whole industry has been able to leave the confines of the beauty parlor and become an independent salon. The services are rendered with such speed and deftness that it is not unusual to be in and out of the nail salon with a complete manicure and pedicure in half an hour. Efficiency-oriented young people have taken over this once tedious service to the client.

In many states, no license is required for nail services. Therefore, there are thousands of available jobs open to new operators. The pay is directly proportional to the operator's agility with the implements and ability to apply artificial tips, wraps, and polish.

Around the New York City area, an operator's income can be as high as $75 to $125 per day with tips included.

Regular beauty salons also employ manicurists and pedicurists. Unlike operators in nail salons, operators in beauty salons rarely have appointments scheduled throughout the day. However, beauty salon operators have the potential to earn good tips because beauty salons generally charge more for their services, and clients are appreciative of the more luxurious treatments they receive in the beauty salons. The nail salon is geared to efficiency first, but both methods have their following.

Manicuring

Many people who have had serious nail problems have discovered that with consistent professional care, nails can become strong, healthy, and attractive. It may be that the nail's being incorrectly filed has caused the weakness and breakage.

You will notice after several trips to the manicurist that the routine is a very exacting one. A professional manicurist trains the nail to grow in a certain manner to strengthen it and to make the nail more attractive to the eye. The end of the nail can be treated so that breakage is kept at a minimum.

One of the advantages of being a manicurist is that your work will not demand that you be on your feet, like other cosmetologists. Instead you can be comfortably seated. Your arms rest on a manicure table, and even when you administer hand and arm massage to a patron, you work gently with no great expenditure of energy. If standing on your feet all day as a hairdresser is too exhausting for you, you might consider specializing in manicuring.

In a busy salon, a manicurist is kept working most of the time. Your tips will depend on your clientele, but the more customers that return to you on a weekly basis, the better your salary will be.

Pedicuring

If you choose to do manicuring only, there is normally enough demand in any beauty or nail salon to keep you busy. But unless you work in a large salon, you will not be able to survive doing just pedicures. Most women who are on their feet for a good portion of the day appreciate the services of a pedicurist. The punishment that feet endure is somewhat counterbalanced by the pedicurist. When toenails are properly clipped, trimmed, filed, and buffed, shoes fit better and blisters are less likely to occur. When toenails are too long, serious damage can occur to the whole foot. People develop incorrect patterns of walking when nails that are too long force feet back and do not allow them to lie flat. It is imperative that the length of toenails be watched, the width of the nail be guided in its growth pattern, and corns, if present, be kept under control. A pedicure is not a luxury. Good nail care is truly a necessity.

After their nails are filed and smooth, some people may want to have them painted. In the summer, or anytime that toes are visible, colored nail polish is a fashion accessory.

SALARIES AND WORKING CONDITIONS

As a manicurist, your weekly salary could be any amount from nothing to $300 depending upon creative talents and your own ability to attract customers. You will have to advise your clients how to protect their nails by wrapping them, how to strengthen the vulnerable ends of long nails, and how a complete plastic nail can shield a badly broken nail until it has a chance to grow out. A manicurist who merely cleans, trims, and polishes nails will earn much less than one who is competent in creatively reconstructing nails.

In New York City, a manicurist may earn as much as $400 a week, plus tips. A pedicurist, who, by the way, makes a higher per-client income, may earn from $15 per hour upward.

You will be able to find work in beauty salons, department stores, barber shops, hotel beauty shops, and specialty salons for nails. There are many new openings yearly for manicurists and pedicurists. It is a profession that takes care, patience, and a genuine interest in a client's well being.

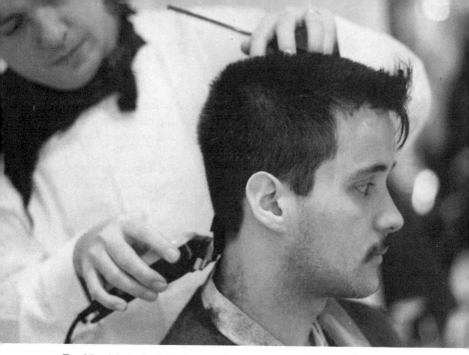

Top: Most jobs in the field of cosmetology are in hair salons. (Glemby International photo) *Bottom*: This beauty consultant works for a cosmetic company. (Mary Kay Cosmetics, Inc. photo)

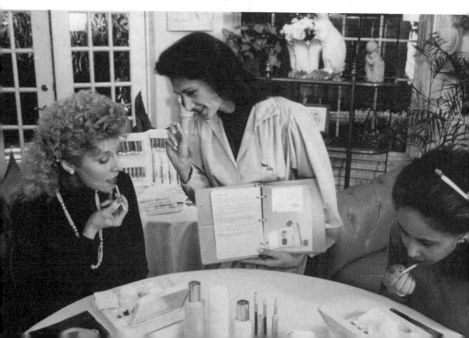

CHAPTER 5

EMPLOYMENT AS A COSMETOLOGIST

You will want to seek employment as a cosmetologist in the most favorable area for your own needs, be they financial, aesthetic, or both. Your cosmetology placement service can help you decide where to apply and will guide you to openings available. Though no one has a crystal ball to predict the future, you must try to foresee the potential for continued success with patrons, both as you begin your job and after you have expanded your clientele. It would be unwise to take a position in an area where you know that a competitor at a more desirable location would be opening soon.

After you get your state certificate, you may want to place your own "position wanted" ad in your local paper and in any city where you might want to work.

Make phone calls to any of the beauty salons, hotels, department stores, or specialty shops where you think that you might like to work. Set up appointments for interviews, and be sure to look neat and well-groomed when you go to the interview.

CHOOSING A PLACE TO WORK

Nursing Homes

There are many places where you can be employed. If you like service work, you may want to work in a hospital or old age home, giving cosmetic services to incapacitated people. Your responsibilities would include shampooing, cutting, manicuring, and pedicuring. Many patients are unable to groom themselves, and your presence would be very needed and appreciated.

Children's Salons

If you really love working with children, there are wonderful positions open for shampooing and cutting children's hair. Many department stores have special shops to cut children's hair in surroundings oriented to their particular needs. In working with children, patience is a must. Many children hate having their hair cut. Even if you try every trick in the world, from hobby horse chair seats to bribes of balloons, it can still be a challenge. But it can pay very well, and parents are grateful.

Beauty Shops

Most jobs in the field of cosmetology are in beauty salons. These salons can be situated anywhere, from the local shopping mall to elegant specialty shops. There are many jobs for general operators and specialists alike. The general employment rate in cosmetology currently seems to be a two-to-one ratio—there are usually two cosmetologists for every one job that is open. So scout your potential area for possible job availability, and allow for time to find a good position. To have the job you desire, you may have to commute a little. Not all cosmetologists are working, or even desire to do so. Statistics are based both on how many cosmetologists are licensed in a particular state and on how many currently are employed in that state. There are always jobs available in service careers, and cosmetology, like all other services, is growing rapidly in certain high-income areas such as New York, Los Angeles, San Francisco, Atlanta, and Chicago. But finding employment can be extremely difficult in areas of lower incomes.

Cruise Lines

If you are interested in a job with travel privileges, you may look into the major cruise lines. There are beauty salons on every luxury liner, and several beauticians are needed for each ship. Manicurists and pedicurists are also needed on shipboard.

There are also openings for facial experts, makeup artists, and barbers. If that particular idea interests you, be sure to list all the possible jobs that you could fill when you apply. Tips are better than average, and benefits are very good. Unless you are working on a cruise ship, you will have all the free time you want while you are in home port. A cruise ship will keep you busy most of the time, as passengers live on board very much as they do in a hotel. You would still have designated free time in each port.

Cosmetic Companies

If you are mainly interested in makeup, your field is wide open. Every major cosmetic company is a potential employer. Apply to several, and get an idea of what will be available at the time you graduate. You may desire to do demonstration work. In this capacity, you would work in the cosmetic company school, where you would be expected to actually demonstrate the cosmetic product at the same time that you show the future sales corps how to apply makeup or cleansing products. There are various other jobs open to the makeup artist. Demonstration is only the beginning, although you could make a very solid career of doing only that. Your job can be as elaborate as your creative capabilities will permit. You could be hired to be a color advisor, and through your own familiarity with shading, shape, texture, and blending, you would work your way up the ladder. Experience is extremely critical here, and your own artistic and creative abilities will come into play as time goes by. With the development of an artist's eye, you may become a makeup specialist.

As you become known in your field, you might want to free-lance. As a freelancer you are your own manager, and you choose your own jobs. You register with an agent in a larger city, and he or she contacts you with clients for your professional services. If you live in a smaller town, word of mouth or your printed business card could bring you jobs. You might find yourself doing makeup for an entire bridal party in a church basement, preparing a face for a local television show, and demonstrating correct makeup to an airline's school all in one week. (There are several states that will permit you to apply makeup only if you are licensed, and then only in a *licensed* place. So once again, check your state's laws first.)

The makeup artist often has fun while he or she is paid very well. Though the top jobs, of course, are very limited, the makeup artists at the most expensive beauty salons and the people who make up the celebrities started out just as you are going to— at the bottom. Any extra art courses that you can take will be helpful. Many hours of practice will also make you more adept at applying makeup.

Many fashionable boutiques hire makeup artists to acquaint their clientele with the latest products and their uses. Even pharmacies have job openings for makeup sales and demonstration. There are many overlapping positions in makeup and sales, and the employer should tell you if any certification or license is required.

As a makeup artist, you could be called to work at a live modeling show, theater, department store, beauty salon, a promotional show, such as a hairdresser's convention or product promotion for television, or almost anywhere in the world where beauty is of interest. On-location work could take you to any country. Catalog work alone could keep you very busy. It takes many years to be in demand as a known makeup artist, but the work is available and your ambition and talents will be your guide.

As a manicurist, you will be able to find work in any beauty salon, specialty shop, hotel, barber shop, department store, nail replacement center, nail sculpting salon, and sometimes on location where nails are to be filmed for a commercial, television show, or film. A note here: It is absolutely critical that any cosmetologist have perfectly trimmed, smooth, clean nails when working on a client's face, head, hands, or body. Sanitary codes strictly dictate cleanliness. Your training in beauty school will have shown you how to follow these codes.

Cosmetic companies usually place help wanted ads, but if you have decided to go into facial work, contact one of the companies directly. You can call or write for an appointment. Tell them about your interests, qualifications, and experience, as well as your schooling and licenses or certifications. Have a professional résumé drawn up to leave with the personnel interviewer. There are many assistantships in large companies, and working as an assistant could be a way for you to reach your final goal.

Barber Shops and Men's Hair Salons

Barber-hairstylists find work in barber shops, unisex shops, hotels, department stores, and specialty shops. There are many small businesses that cut men's hair. A visit to inquire about future employment may be your best course. There are barbers who work on men, women, and even children. Your work as a unisex stylist would permit you to practice anywhere that a cosmetology license is not required.

As a specialist in any area, such as coloring, wiggery, shampooing, or hairweaving, you are limited to working in those salons that offer the particular specialty that you are qualified to practice.

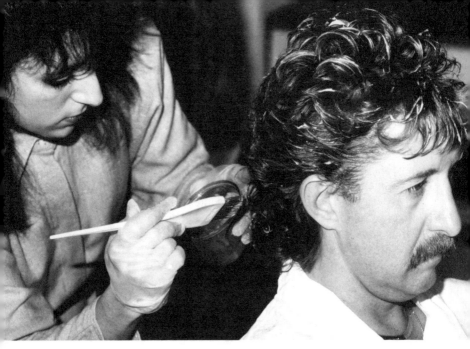

Top: Experienced hair colorists are in demand by both male and female customers. (L'Oreal International Salon Institute photo) *Bottom* : Manicurists and pedicurists often find employment in beauty salons. (Pittsburgh Beauty Academy photo)

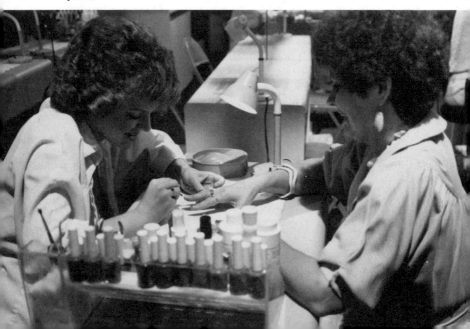

CHAPTER 6

THE BEAUTY SALON

According to recent statistics, one out of every two licensed cosmetologists owns his or her own beauty salon. This means that there are wide open horizons for your advancement in the field. The smallest of these establishments requires a skeleton staff that does many jobs, but there are beauty salon franchises that can accommodate thousands of cosmetologists in their shops.

Every position in a beauty salon is important to the smooth running of the entire business. Like any professional operation, everything must appear neat, clean, efficient, and pleasant. Patrons want to feel that staff members know what they are doing. If things look too relaxed or sloppy, your patron will not feel confident that you will be able to accomplish a professional job. Many people are very fearful of trusting a hairdresser after a bad experience. Your place of work should encourage and support the benefits of good grooming, not fill the patron with concern.

BEAUTY SALON JOBS

Receptionist

The receptionist is a nonlicensed person who welcomes the patron, acknowledges the appointment, and shows the patron where to go. The receptionist also answers the phone, sets up appointments, and lets the operators know what time the patrons will arrive. The pay for this position is normally minimum wage, unless the duties are not limited to the aforementioned.

Checkroom Attendant

The checkroom attendant takes your coat and gives you a dressing gown to put on. Various chemicals could harm your clothing, and for that reason you are asked to change from your upper clothing into a loose fitting smock. Hair tends to cling to clothing, and it is extremely irritating to the skin. Wearing a smock will keep cut hair from getting on your clothes. The checkroom attendant often receives a very small salary, or none at all, and must live on tips alone. If the checkroom is a concession, the attendant may be paid a portion of the tips and no salary. All payment should be clearly spelled out beforehand.

Beautician's Assistant

The beautician's assistant is usually an apprentice who holds a state license. Requirements vary from state to state. An apprentice usually is paid a small amount while polishing his or her skills as a stylist, hair colorist, or permanent wave specialist. The beautician's assistant does shampooing, scalp massage, roller holding, blow-drying, removes rollers, and brushes hair off the patron for final clean-up. An assistant does not cut hair or do any actual hairstyling, but observes the hairstylist and receives on-the-job training. This is a very good way to make a name for yourself in a better salon where the highest salaries and tips are earned. As an assistant you could expect to be paid around $90, plus tips, per week. Some salons will not pay that much, but the education you get as an assistant is similar to advanced education. And the more that a hairstylist knows, the higher his or her salary.

Hair Coloring and Permanents

Hair colorists are much in demand, as most women at some time or other dye their hair. There are several types of hair color. Temporary colors are called tints and can be shampooed out. For the patron who is not ready for the dramatic leap to hair dyeing, a rinse or tint is the answer. A color rinse is great for making grey hair blend or to give highlights. It is not an overall solid color, as is dye. Hair dyeing and bleaching can take many years of training. A thorough understanding of chemicals is critical. Patch tests must be done on every patron to check for possible allergic reaction. The hair colorist does semipermanent and permanent haircolors, hennas, highlighting, retouching, lightening, toning, frosting, streaking, tipping, and hair painting. All of these different processes take many years to master. Assistants work alongside experienced hair colorists to learn the craft of hair coloring.

In dyeing hair, timing is of the utmost importance. Even though hair colorists use timers, they must concentrate their attention on the patrons. Serious damage could occur to the hair if the dye is left on too long. Hair colorists earn very good salaries, anywhere from $400 per week upward, plus tips, depending on their particular place of business.

Permanent waving, hair pressing, and chemical hair relaxing are all specialties. The size of the salon and the volume of business will dictate how many of these professionals are employed in a salon. Any specialist is able to command a salary of at least $400 to $550 a week. Again, it depends on whether or not he or she is paid a straight salary, a commission, or a combination of the two. Tips are usually excellent in any good hair salon, and the more specialized the service, the higher the tips.

Manicurists

Manicurists and pedicurists also have their places of employment in beauty salons. Patrons usually have these services done while their hair is being dried. Pedicurists normally work in a sectioned-off area to give the patron more privacy. In larger salons, these services are well rewarded with tips. Salaries vary from a per-patron percentage to a straight salary of around $175 a week. This is not a clear-cut area, as many manicurists earn a salary that changes, sometimes from week to week. It seems to depend on special patrons who come back time and again.

Makeup and Facial Specialists

Makeup artists and facial experts might be employed in a beauty parlor, probably a very large place of business offering full services to the patrons. Services in this type of establishment would include leg waxing, wig styling, and even salespeople demonstrating products to patrons.

Hairstylists

The most important and most recognized people in any beauty parlor are hairstylists. These men and women are highly skilled and well-trained experts in cutting hair in particular hairstyles. Haircutting is the most difficult part of handling hair. Hair can have different textures such as wiry, slippery, thick, fine, coarse, limp, and curly. Hair is a challenge to control, and haircuts train hair to lie in a desired manner. Top stylists can and do earn salaries commensurate with their abilities. Haircuts alone in New York can cost up to $100. The average hairstylist earns about $60 per cut, plus tips. Arrangements vary from employer to employer. If you are working for yourself, the sky is the limit for your potential income.

Other Positions

There are other positions in the beauty salon that do not require state licensing. These jobs entail handling supplies. Stockpersons and laundry and cleaning personnel are all necessary for a functioning shop. The person who sees to the smooth running of it all is the manager. This person is responsible for the coordination of hiring and firing. He or she also makes up the employee work schedules, schedules vacations, orders paychecks and uniforms, places advertisements, orders supplies and sales merchandise, and acts as peacemaker, should any disagreements arise in the shop. A manager's thorough knowledge of beauty professions and the business workings of the salon can guarantee the success of the shop. A manager's salary normally corresponds to his or her responsibilities. If the salon is particularly large and complex, the salary will be excellent.

Retail Sales

Retail selling in beauty salons has become a new way to add to the income of the shop itself and to the incomes of the operators, manicurists, pedicurist, and wig stylist.

Most of the more famous salons promote their own cosmetics and hair products. Depending on how large the retail aspect of their business is, many salons actually have a salesperson in the employ of the salon. If there is no specific salesperson, the operator who recommends the special hair treatment or shampoo will receive commission on the sale. The beauty salon, of course, covers its cost and a small commission as well. Many specialists sell almost all of the creams, lotions, packs, scrubs, astringents, cleansers, and makeup that they use in the salon itself. Once the client is introduced to the product and is given instruction on how to apply it, he or she can do the same service at home. A shampoo specialist usually recommends the type of shampoo and rinse needed for a customer's particular scalp, and more often than not, these products are sold in the beauty shop. Product lines have been expanded to include the salon's own hairdryers, combs, styling brushes, and even bags large enough to carry all the products.

Manicuring specialties and different products used to make the nails stronger and keep them from looking unkempt are also sold in beauty salons. These creams are applied daily to supplement the once-a-week visit to the manicurist.

Wigs and postiches are often sold in beauty salons as well as all the required accessories, such as wig spray, carrier cases, brushes, and even clips and bows. These items can increase the income of the salon tremendously. And if a salon services wigs and postiches, it would be a mistake not to sell them. The profit is very high on both natural and synthetic pieces.

Most women and men who have just come from a hairstylist's care and look their best will assume that part of the result is the product the hairstylist used. The psychology of selling the product right there is very powerful. If you suggest to your client that she or he go out and purchase the items that you have used in their treatment, chances are small that they will even remember the name of the product, let alone the procedure. Having the products accessible is only good business and good treatment for your client. Many salon patrons feel that it was not their weekly visit to the hairstylist that was expensive but all those irresistible little goodies that added up to a very sizable income for the salon owner.

CHAPTER 7

FACIAL SALONS AND SKIN CARE

THE NEED FOR FACIAL SPECIALISTS

Facial specialists have come into their own in the last few years. This service was known chiefly in the salons of Europe and Japan. Salons in the United States are catching up, and job opportunities for estheticians are now quite common in any community. The need for facial and skin care services accompanies the products that are used for facial manipulations and massage. This service was used only by the very wealthy until about ten years ago. This luxurious, pleasurable treatment has now become well known, and costs range from $30 to $75 for about an hour's work. Facial care specialists often earn generous tips for providing this luxurious service with its aura of glamour.

Too much of any natural element can guarantee a skin of leather consistency. Exposed skin will form a heavy and darker texture to protect itself from further damage. The sad thing about damaged skin is that the damage is more often than not permanent. Skin dried out from too much sun will never be soft and delicate again. We are still learning what permanent damage the sun can cause. We now know that a little direct sunlight is vital, but it must be acquired gradually. If our faces were not exposed, we would not need highly specialized techniques to protect this vulnerable area. Grime and dirt attack our faces and hands. But even hands have tougher skin than faces. Not only that, but gloves and mittens at least partially protect hands during many times of the year. So what appears to be one of the most delicate of skin areas is expected to meet all kinds of weather and remain attractive, young, and as unlined as possible.

There are many ways moisture can be retained in the skin, facial muscles toned and exercised, and dirt and excessive oil removed from the face. The specialist who is most knowledgeable in this field will not only have a cosmetologist's license but will have had several weeks of intensive schooling in highly skilled techniques.

Even if a person is not troubled with any particular skin problems and has the luck to have absolutely radiant skin, the services of a skin specialist can ward off potential trouble through skin analysis, helping the skin to stay as young as physically possible.

Skin care is also known as *esthetics.* If someone specializes in the care of the skin, he or she could be known as a cosmetician, a skin care analyst, an esthetician, a skin therapist, or a skin specialist. When you are looking for work, you could conceivably be listed as any of these and still work exclusively with the face.

There are several ways to break into the facial care world. But first you will have to complete your state boards so that you will be a licensed cosmetologist. In some states you will go directly into facial specialty work without further instruction. Some states require that you obtain a specialty certificate. In New York, for example, you need both the certificate and the state license to land a good job with higher pay and more opportunity for advancement. But you can get a job doing facials in a beauty salon with just your state licensing. In general, if you want to specialize, try to get as much instruction as you can afford from as highly recognized an authority as possible. Education is the fastest and surest way up the professional ladder. One word of recommendation from a well-known figure in your chosen field can be extremely valuable.

EDUCATION FOR FACIAL SPECIALISTS

Your basic skin care work will be covered in beauty school training. You will learn how to manually cleanse, manipulate, and massage the skin. You will have a little skin analysis, some anatomy and physiology pertaining to the skin, and a brief course on diseases of the skin. It is critical that you understand all the possible disorders of the skin for health precautions. You should also know your own limitations in being able to determine whether a minor case of acne can be corrected or whether a doctor's advice is needed. You must be able to identify a bump or lump on or beneath the skin's surface before you apply anything to the client's skin. It could be a harmless fatty cyst or something infectious that could be contagious to you or other patrons.

You will want to familiarize yourself with the skin's functions and conditions so you will be able to advise your client on preventive or corrective measures. Most clients will have similar problems. Many younger people have skin that tends to be too oily and middle-aged, too dry. It is pleasurable to have the skin manipulated at any age, and a variety of massages are indicated by skin types. Some massage is for relaxing, and some is for stimulating. The muscles of the face benefit from the effects of massage. Tensions and stress show on the face more than on any other part of the body. Massage can reduce stressful feelings by causing tension to disappear. Tight muscles can also be therapeutically relaxed with heat and light. Some techniques employ several processes in one treatment. You might have electric massage (stimulation) with heat, or after an application of an abrasive cream, steam might be prescribed. Chemical reactions speed up with the addition of heat. If the opposite treatment is called for, astringents cool and close pores. A skilled skin specialist can teach you how to take the best care of your skin. Cleaning your type of skin can be more complex than just soap and water, and many soaps dry delicate facial skin. Even if you have plenty of oil now, you could be harming your skin by not giving it the proper care it needs.

GETTING AN EDUCATION AND FINDING A JOB

Scientific skin care is now available in most large cities and in many smaller ones. As it is a comparatively new career field in the United States, you may have a little difficulty locating a school that specializes in facial care. Look under "esthetics school" in your yellow pages. If you do not find any listing of that nature, write to your state board requesting information on specialty schools. You might try calling a major city telephone operator for a skin care school listing.

Most states require one hundred to two hundred hours for licensure after state cosmetology licensing. Some states also require a high school education before you enroll in skin care school.

The approximate cost for a facial care program is about $600 for four weeks of instruction. There is also a complete program for makeup which does not require state licensing in all states. And you can also practice the art of esthetics without a beauty school background.

One particular school has branches in many large cities across the United States. The woman who manages the New York branch says that no one had even heard of this specialty where she came from in England. So if facial care seems like an interesting career possibility to you, do not be discouraged by its apparent inaccessibility. Facial schools do exist in the major cities, and you should be able to find one by checking the yellow pages.

Two states already have made a distinction between a cosmetology license and a facial care license, Louisiana and Massachusetts. Upon completion of four hundred hours of schooling in facial care you could be a fully qualified specialist in these two states. You would still have to pass your exams but not the extended ones set up by the cosmetology boards. Your work would be restricted to facial care and makeup.

In California there is a special course of six hundred hours that permits you to apply for certification and registration as a cosmetician. Like a skin care or facial specialist, you are permitted to give facials; apply makeup; give skin care; remove

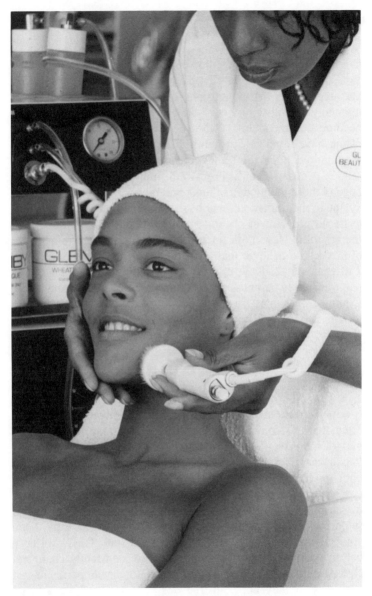

Job opportunities for facial specialists are rapidly increasing as more customers demand this glamorous service. (Glemby International photo)

hair by depilatory, waxing, or tweezing; and apply false eyelashes. You are licensed to apply preparations to the neck, bust, arms, and upper body. Massaging and cleaning skin by machine and manually are also services you are permitted to perform. To become a cosmetician in California, you must be seventeen years of age, have completed the tenth grade, and received the minimum six hundred hours of training from an approved cosmetology school. A cosmetician is prohibited from practicing any services beyond those mentioned in this paragraph.

Due to the limited number of strictly facial salons, there seems to be no problem in placing certified graduates. Salons contact the school in New York for recommendations, and the manager of this school believes that all of the graduates find work. About 250 students graduate each year. Incomes start at about $175 per week, plus commissions, or a straight salary of about $250. Commission comes from volume of customers or products sold to the customer. Facial salons often carry their own line of cleansing products and cosmetics.

OPENING A FACIAL SALON

After a student completes the facial care course, he or she often opens a salon. If you start with your own salon, the beginning may be a bit rough until you have established your own clientele. It is a very lucrative business that can be run by a small staff until you have more patrons.

If you open a skin care salon, you will then need a state license for cosmetology and a certificate for skin care. If you open a salon that dispenses only cosmetics and you demonstrate them, you no longer need a license in New York state. Check all laws before opening a salon, because laws are constantly changing. New state boards make new laws, and what was pertinent last year may or may not hold true this year. If you open a facial salon in Louisiana or Massachusetts, you will need only the facial course and no license from the state. If all this seems terribly complicated, it is because there are no national standards, and each state governs its own cosmetology businesses. It is not likely that you will practice in many states during your lifetime, but if you do move around, the sad truth is that you will have to take a practical and a written test every time you cross over a state line.

TEACHING FACIAL SPECIALTY SKILLS

Facial specialists may also find jobs as instructors in schools teaching facial care. If you are interested in teaching facial technique, you are required to have three years of experience in the field and the required teaching courses offered at the college level. A separate teaching license must be obtained from the state at a cost of about $500. These are the requirements of New York state.

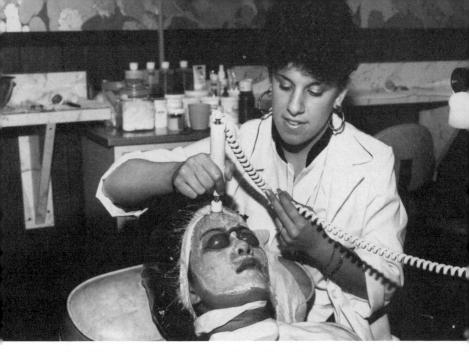

Top: Makeup specialists analyze their clients' skin and help them develop a cleansing regimen. (Pittsburgh Beauty Academy photo) *Bottom*: A variety of cosmetic products is used to blend and highlight facial features. (Glemby International photo)

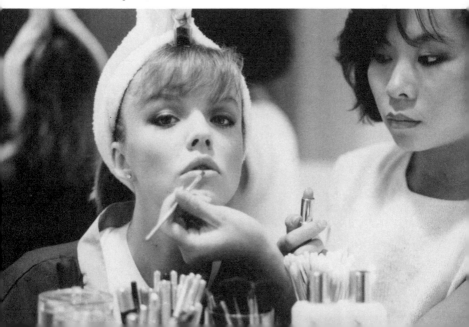

CHAPTER 8

MAKEUP

Makeup artists are highly recognized today as respected professionals in the beauty industry. The demand has shifted from making up actors and actresses to demonstrating to the public how to correctly apply the thousands of cosmetic products that confront the baffled purchaser in every department store in the world. With plastic surgery, a whole new aspect of makeup has emerged, and the makeup artist has dozens of clever tricks and illusions to communicate to the client.

The first responsibility that a makeup specialist has to his or her patrons is to analyze their skin and advise them how to clean it correctly. Everyone has a different skin type, and the balance between the skin's natural oils and what is applied externally is important. If you have skin that lacks moisture and oils, you will follow a program designed to save the resources that are already in scarce supply in your body. If your skin is very oily, it is unlikely that all areas of your face are in that condition. So a specialist's analysis is a form of advice to the patron, and he or she must know the signs of dry or oily areas. When a specialist sees flakes of dry skin around a client's nose, for example, he or she should realize that those dead skin cells need to be removed so that the underlying cells can breathe. Contrary to belief, dry skin that is flaking does not indicate lack of oils, but the opposite. Stimulation to that area is needed so that dead cells are naturally sloughed off.

SKIN CARE

Makeup is a profession in which communication is vital. It is important for makeup specialists to clearly explain what problems they recognize in a customer's skin and how a beauty program is to be followed for best results. There are many people with beautiful faces whose skin was not so trouble-free when they used improper care. Cleansing the face is a top priority. Cleansers come in liquid, cream, and even bar shapes. A combination of several of these cleansers is usually used to achieve really clean skin. Someone who lives in a city has more dirt to battle and needs more help in deep cleaning. Scrubs and pore cleansers are a necessity for normal or oily skin. Dry skin needs protection from the elements as well, usually in the form of remoisturizers.

Astringents are applied to every skin type to close pores. All preparations come in varying strengths, and your job will include understanding every type of skin's needs.

Unfortunately, the cleansing procedure removes needed oils as well as surface oil and dirt. Astringents also remove remaining surface oil, and this must be replaced by applying moisturizers. There are various ways to remoisturize the skin. The most delicate, the lightest creams, are the most easily accepted by the skin. Even if a person has a good supply of natural oils, there will be areas depleted of oils. Your professional eye will have to quickly analyze any problems and advise the patron of the most efficient way to deal with them. Your ability to save patrons time in their daily cleansing routine is very important. If they have to allot more time than is practical in their daily routine, they may not complete it. If so, the skin will suffer. If an individual takes preventions when he or she is young, he or she can maintain young, healthy, supple skin well past middle age.

COLOR

The amount of color in a face also can be changed with makeup. There are two ways in which color can work to improve appearance. The first is by altering the contour of the bones of the face. Every face is unequal in its two halves. Your job would be to see what is uneven and shade or add color as the fault dictates. One of the highest paid cosmetic models today has a notoriously uneven face. A breakdown of her features actually showed the two halves of her face to be unequal by an inch and a half. Most faces have much more subtle inequalities. This model supposedly was given a choice modeling contract because ordinary people could relate to her imperfect beauty and were more inclined to buy the company's cosmetics.

The second way in which color can be used to correct facial defects is in concealing certain "bad colors." If dark circles, sallowness, or ruddiness dominate a face, careful selection of concealers and foundations can alter them. Small scars or blemishes also can be covered by concealers. The old method of covering the entire face with heavy makeup is not only extremely unattractive but very bad for the skin's ability to breathe. A touch of color is enough to achieve the effect of natural good looks. Remember that you are teaching someone how to improve his or her skin's color, so explanations are necessary. Many women buy a product without the slightest idea how it should be used. Really make an effort to explain what you are doing in terms that your patron will understand and remember. Few ladies can afford the services of a trained makeup advisor every time they apply their cosmetics, so your job is to relay all pertinent information in simple terms. Many people who have looked really lovely after a professional application of makeup have later been very unsure when it is their turn to apply it to themselves. Experience is essential, and encouragement is part of your responsibility to your patron. Makeup is an art that many women have cleverly taught themselves through guidance from makeup people. Not all of us are gifted with a steady hand, let alone the artist's eye, so practice and patience are essential.

There are wide varieties of cosmetic products used to blend and highlight different facial features. The eyes are the most expressive facial feature, and because they are often smaller than we would like them to be, much concentration is put into eye makeup. Eye color can be enhanced and made more vibrant by adding eyeliner or eye shadow. The iris (colored part of the eye) is affected by any color that it reflects. By clever use of shadows, eyes can be made to look closer together, farther apart, rounder, and larger. Great skill is needed to bring about these corrections, but with a light touch, you will be able to develop that talent in due time.

Sheen or high gloss are other cosmetic additives that can create special effects. Where a surface is shiny, it will appear to protrude and call attention to itself. This is usually a texture appearance that is applied to cheeks, lips, or even eyelids. The skin on different parts of the face varies greatly. Look at the difference between the surface of the lips and the tightly stretched skin on the bridge of the nose. These differences will dictate not only the texture of the makeup to be applied but also the quantity. Usually the rule of thumb is to use a small amount with a light touch.

The overall look is the final goal. Nothing should stand out. The eyes, eyebrows, eyelids, cheeks, and lips should be highlighted, and the rest of the face should be a perfect, unflawed background to set off the features.

EDUCATION

There are several places where you can receive instruction to do makeup. Many cosmetic companies train and develop talents through continued guidance and instruction, especially as their new products come out. Practice is the key word, and you will be expected to blend old products with new ones in actual makeup work. Many cosmetic companies provide schooling taught by their own staff at no cost to you.

Sometimes the schooling is as little as a week in length, and you are expected to gain your experience on the job. You obviously cannot learn makeup in a week, so observing the more experienced makeup person's technique is invaluable. You usually are asked

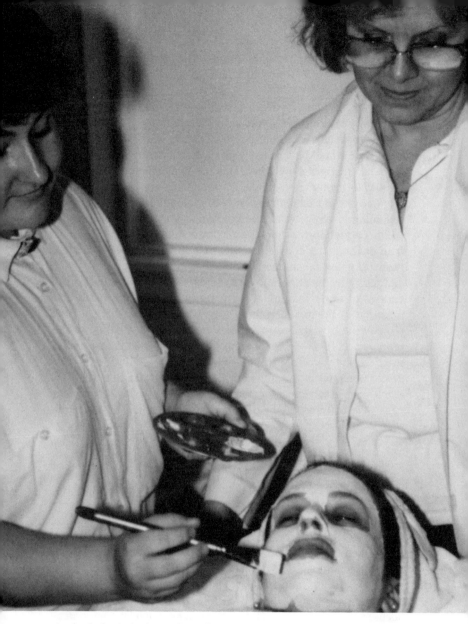

A school of esthetics is one place where students can receive instruction to do makeup. (Dallas Institute of Aesthetics and Body Therapy, photo by Johnnie Parker)

to do very minimal work in actual application of makeup until you really start to have a feel for it.

You could also take your training in a school of esthetics. There the course would be whatever the state required. The one in New York has a program of thirty-five hours, and the tuition is currently $200. No license is required for graduates unless they wish to work in a state demanding one. In states that require licenses, schooling in cosmetics may be taken as a special course, or the whole cosmetology school training may be required.

In one makeup class, the curriculum included makeup design, transformation techniques, application of false eyelashes, color and harmony, and special work for day and evening. Two other courses of thirty-five hours each were offered in advanced and theatrical makeup. The tuition was $250. Most of the students already held state certification, even though it was not a prerequisite. If you do not obtain a license, you could be prevented from working where a license is required. This could limit your career potential in this competitive, but very satisfying, field. To reach your greatest career potential, you may want to complete your state cosmetology boards.

LICENSING

Cosmetology boards for makeup are a requirement in many states. In most states, a small number of school hours are set aside for the strict pursuit of skin analysis, corrective or complete makeup, or application of false eyelashes. You will notice that all of these require actually touching the patron, the point on which laws differ. In some states, you cannot touch the patron without a license, and in other states, as long as the service is performed only on the skin's surface (makeup, electrology), a license is not required. There is no consistency in the states' prohibitions. Certain services that are considered purely cosmetic in some states are regulated by medical boards in others.

JOBS IN MAKEUP

The places where you might seek employment after you are a makeup person could be almost anywhere. Department stores, drugstores, cosmetic company demonstrations on various locations, beauty salons, specialty shops. promotionals, beauty shows, modeling shows, theaters, television, and movies all offer jobs for makeup specialists. Most jobs available are in the sales area of cosmetic companies. This is often the springboard for many career jobs in cosmetics.

The qualifications for finding a job in makeup include finger dexterity, patience, a good eye for facial structure, a clear understanding of colors and how to create them (remember that skin has its own color—it is not a clean white canvas), and a genuine interest in helping people to look better.

Pay scales vary greatly depending on which position you take. But starting pay is almost never below $200 a week. In large cities, pay would more than likely be over $225. Your decision to work on commission and salary, or just salary, will affect your income, too.

Makeup is a rapidly expanding field, and hundreds of jobs occur with each new cosmetic company. You have a wide open field from which to choose. You may select full- or part-time work, sales, demonstration, or even door-to-door sales. There is an opening in the cosmetic job market that could very likely satisfy you.

Makeup work has continued to be an area of immense growth. There is hardly any area in the world today where you cannot find diversified cosmetics from many companies. In New York City alone, millions of dollars are spent annually on cosmetic products. And thousands of jobs are created from this demand.

Makeup jobs are not found only in large cities. New products are distributed in the most remote corners of the earth. And as these products are distributed, they create jobs.

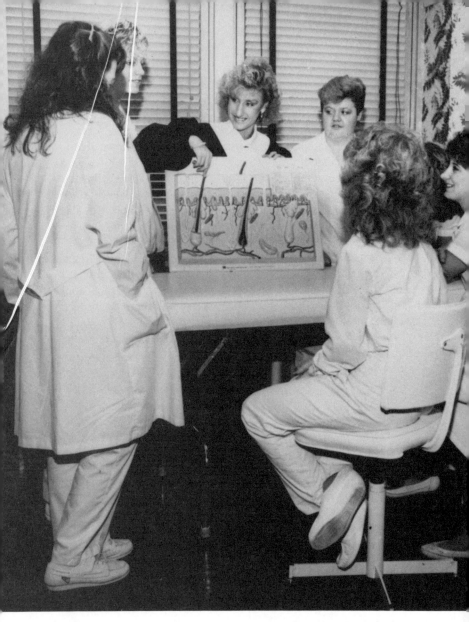

Students receive technical instruction on electrolysis, generally considered to be the safest method of permanent hair removal. (Pittsburgh Beauty Academy photo)

CHAPTER 9

ELECTROLOGISTS, EPILATIONISTS, AND THERMOLOGISTS

The removal of unwanted hair is done by an electrologist or an epilationist. The actual procedure is called electrolysis, which involves permanently removing hair by removing the hair follicle with an electrical current. You may want to make an appointment with a professional operator if you think that you may be interested in a career in this area of cosmetology. The schools that teach electrolysis are quite frequently run by salespeople who sell the electrical equipment that is used in this process. Some beauty schools do teach electrology, but since there is no licensing required in many states, there are few schools that offer the course in their curriculum.

Our society dictates who should have hair growth, where it should grow, and even how much hair is socially acceptable. Long underarm hair with sleeveless clothing is not considered proper grooming in most social circles. Even nostril hair is groomed with scissors by a barber. You cannot have electrolysis on nostril hairs or hairs that grow on moles and warts. Your electrologist can advise you on other areas not suitable for electrolysis. If you are diabetic or have a pacemaker, it is advisable to have medical clearance before you have electrolysis.

As an electrologist, you learn how to insert a very fine needle or wire into a hair follicle. The needle (contrary to popular belief) never punctures the skin. It is merely inserted in the natural opening of the hair follicle. A gentle electrical current is then applied to the papilla (hair cell). As a result of this process, the papilla dies and the hair is then removed with a tweezer. An electrologist works with a large magnifying glass that has a light around its circumference. There is a certain amount of eye strain in this job because electrologists must concentrate on one hair at a time. After you build up your finger dexterity, you will be able to remove many hairs in a few minutes. The needle is held in one hand while you spread or stretch the skin gently with the other hand. While looking through the magnifying glass, you will be able to quickly guide the needle into the hair follicle.

EDUCATION

Electrolysis is generally considered to be the safest method of permanent hair removal if performed by a qualified electrologist with up-to-date electric equipment. Therefore it is critical that you attend a good school of electrolysis. In the state of New York, you will need to attend classes to receive your certificate. The typical school requires 120 hours of work. The curriculum consists of lectures, actual clinic work with electrolysis machines and patrons, and testing. The minimum age is usually eighteen, with no formal schooling required. There is usually no language barrier problem, as the work is of a practical nature. For instance, if you could speak no French and your patrons spoke only French, you would still be permitted to perform electrolysis on them. The only problem might be quoting fees or explaining the actual process if the patron wants to know how electrolysis works. But strictly speaking, you would not have to talk to the patron, only serve him or her. The current price of tuition at a school of electrology is around $1,000 for fifteen eight-hour days. There are evening courses and part-time courses, but you could conceivably have your certificate after three weeks of concentrated schooling.

LICENSING

Laws on electrology differ greatly from state to state. In Massachusetts, for example, 1,100 hours are required prior to taking a state board exam in order to practice electrolysis. In California, an electrology course of five hundred hours taught by an established cosmetology or electrology school must be completed before you can apply for state registration and licensure. Also, the age limit is seventeen, and a twelfth-grade education is a prerequisite for taking the course. So you can see laws are drastically different in the field of electrolysis. In New York you could actually be setting up your own practice in a month's time, while in Massachusetts, you would still be a student after eight months. You will want to consider the time needed to complete a course before you enter a program. You also must realize that if you do decide to take a course in New York and then move to a state with more stringent education requirements, you may find that you have to go back to school and start all over again.

FINDING A JOB

When you graduate from electrology school, you will be able to find work in certain specialty shops, department stores, or your own private salon, if you want to set one up. Unlike the other career possibilities I have discussed (with the possible exception of facial and skin care work), electrologists most often work for themselves. The equipment is minimal. A short wave machine, a couch or a hydraulic chair, and something comfortable for the operator to sit on, magnifying lamps, needles and needle sterilizer, tweezers, and a few antiseptic lotions will be all you need. At a cost of under $6,000 you could be in business for yourself! This is obviously a perfect job for someone who wants to be his or her own boss. Your time is your own, and the average hourly charge for electrolysis can be anywhere from $30 to $75 depending on your area of the country.

Insurance costs for an independent electrologist in New York state are about $125 annually. This fee is so reasonable because there seem to be few malpractice suits.

The field of electrology is wide open for earning. Large numbers of electrologists are not available, and the procedure of removing hair electrically is very time consuming. There are therefore plenty of job opportunities in this necessary and rewarding field. There are many people who have never heard of electrology, and with a little advertising and word-of-mouth praise from your patrons, you might easily establish a career for yourself in a very short time.

To help you learn more about electrolysis, there are several nonprofit organizations exclusively for electrologists. These groups are dedicated to the betterment of the profession, and most actively practicing electrologists are members.

One last word about the actual process of electrically removing hair. It is not painful, but because people have different tolerance levels, some people feel a slight discomfort in more sensitive areas, such as the upper lip. Legs are probably the least sensitive. Patrons who have been treated are usually extremely pleased. Facial hair can make a woman feel far less than feminine, and after all, the main purpose of all cosmetics is to make you your most attractive self.

CHAPTER 10

WIGS, HAIRPIECES, AND HAIRWEAVING

Hair loss has unfortunately become more prevalent as people suffer from chemotherapy, hormone imbalances, and loss due to genetic traits. For many years, hairpieces or wigs were the only possible solutions. Today those suffering from hair loss are offered a choice between hair replacement by adding hair (hairweaving) or a hairpiece. Both processes are quite expensive, and the client will need your professional care for either choice. Hairweaving costs anywhere from $300 to $6000 for the basic work in which hair add-ons are sewn or woven into the client's own existing hair. Then as the natural hair grows out, the add-on hair "grows" out with it. This needs monthly maintenance that runs between $25 and $30. Hairweaving is used as much for enhancing length and volume as for replacing hair.

CHOOSING A WIG

There are two kinds of hair available for wigs, natural and synthetic. A natural wig made of real human hair is the first choice. Human hair used in wigs and hairpieces is chemically boiled to remove the color. Then it is dyed to match a color wheel that gives a precise choice to the patron. Each wig or hairpiece is referred to by a certain number on the color wheel.

The wig must be carefully fitted to the patron's head. If it is too large, it can actually be shrunk by applying hot or warm water to the cap and leaving it to dry on a block smaller than the patron's head. Tucks also can be taken in the cap of the wig to make it the correct size. A new kind of wig has strips of hair held together by elastic. This wig is lighter and lets air reach the scalp because the hair is not a solid mass, unlike the traditional style.

The other kind of wig is made of synthetic hair. This type of wig has its limitations, and synthetic hair often is used in less expensive wigs. Modacrylic fibers are supposedly so cleverly used now that synthetic wigs can look very natural. Of course the actual construction of the wig itself can dictate the quality of the wig. Hand-tied wigs are the best quality, while machine-made ones are less desirable. Some wigs are made using both methods and are considered to be serviceable as well as ornamental. The hand-tied European wig is the most expensive, and the machine-stitched, synthetic fiber wig is the least expensive.

The cost of cleaning the two types relates to the original cost of the wig. The less expensive synthetic wig can be washed in ordinary shampoo and rinsed in water. The natural hair wig is cleaned in a fluid similar to dry cleaning fluid. This fluid is dangerous and must be used in a ventilated area.

Because the care of natural hair wigs is so extensive, the cost is much higher than for a synthetic wig. The natural hair must be conditioned, as natural oils must be cleaned out of the wig along with dirt. Gentle care will guarantee a long life to a real hair wig. It can even be dyed, unlike the synthetic wig.

Hairpieces come in varying sizes and lengths. Women use them for special effects, to give more height or weight to their own hair, or to fill in sparse areas. Hairpieces can be made of artificial or natural hair, machine made or hand tied.

WORKING AS A WIG STYLIST

The job of the wig stylist is to fit, clean, cut, style, and comb out wigs and hairpieces. Packaging the wig in a carrier may also be a duty, as many women never come to the wig stylist, and the stylist must pack and send the wig back to the customer.

If a wig stylist works in a beauty salon, he or she may need a license as a cosmetologist. Often a wig specialist certificate is adequate to work on wigs in salons, department stores, specialty shops, wig shops, or costume departments. State health codes set strict standards for wig handlers. No wig is permitted to touch another wig, and all wigs must be handled so that they are not contaminated by anything that touches them. The block that the wig rests on, the pins that hold it, and the rollers, clips, brushes, or combs that may come in contact with it must all be carefully sanitized.

Wig styling is covered in the New York state licensing for cosmetologists. This permits the wig stylist to actually work on the wig or hairpiece while it is on the patron. Not all wig stylists need to touch the patron, and each stylist has to decide whether he or she needs that extra licensing. If a person is merely selling wigs in a department store, it is highly unlikely that any certification would be required in any state, though he or she may wish to combine actual hairpiece work and wig styling. The particular question of who must be licensed for wig work seems to be undecided. The answer seems to depend on who a stylist is working for, where he or she is working, and if he or she has to touch the client.

SALARIES

Pay scale in the field of wig styling varies. A wig specialist usually receives a commission from the salon for each wig, plus tips. If you work only on the wig and never see the customer, tips would obviously not amount to much. If you are running your own wiggery where you are personally measuring the patron, acquiring, selecting, or recommending wigs (or even making them), and fitting, cutting, and servicing, then your income could be quite substantial.

Your actual salary would also depend greatly on where you are working. People in certain areas of the country find wigs more acceptable and more of a necessity than in others. Large cities are where you would sell and service the greatest number of wigs and hairpieces. Most show business and theater personalities need wigs and own several postiches, toupees, or full wigs.

SELLING HAIRPIECES TO MEN

Men use hairpieces as much or even more than women. In large cities, there are full-page advertisements for hairpieces for men who are balding. Toupees are mentioned briefly here, as they are similar to, but not quite the equivalent of, the postiche for a woman, and you may or may not need licensing in your particular state to handle toupees. It all depends on the laws that cover your state's barbering codes and if hairpieces are regulated under your state's law. In New York City, licensing is needed, as measurements for wigs require touching the patron, the deciding factor. Men's hairpieces are not regulated by cosmetology boards. So though it is highly unlikely that if you work as a cosmetologist you would be doing men's hairpieces, you might be employed in a unisex salon where the question may arise. It is your job to be able to advise your patron, and you should be able to recommend a reliable men's hair care professional.

Hairweaving is performed on as many men as women clients. A customer should be advised of all possibilities before investing in either type of hair replacement.

CHAPTER 11

OWNING YOUR OWN BEAUTY SALON

Current statistics show that half of the working licensed cosmetologists (about 250,000 operators) own and work in their own salons. The greatest number of these are hairstylists. These statistics indicate that advancement in the field of cosmetology involves owning your own salon. The obvious attraction is that you will be your own boss and you will reap more of the profits. Drawbacks are financial responsibilities if the business does not succeed.

Salon owners can earn a salary of between $50,000 and $100,000 annually, depending upon the salon's location and the number of steady clients.

When you are enrolled in cosmetology school, it is very possible that you will have several hours of instruction in owning and managing a beauty salon. In New York state, about fifty hours are devoted to this area in the private beauty school curriculum. Astute planning is of the utmost importance as many complications can develop in trying to coordinate a project of this size. The tiniest salon with area to service two patrons at a time will have all the major problems of a larger one. The difference will be the dispersal of responsibility among the larger staff in a bigger salon.

Before you start your salon, check all of the state codes and local laws that regulate owning and running your own salon. You will be responsible for everything, even if you do have a manager and a very competent staff. Ultimately, as the owner, you are responsible to the state and, of course, to all of your salon's patrons, whether you actually work on the person or one of your employees does. You will be responsible for insurance coverage, rental payments, salaries, hiring, firing, accounting, paying taxes on the business, and purchasing all the supplies. If you do not want to handle the day-to-day operations of your salon, you can delegate these jobs to a manager-operator who is qualified to manage a salon. This person should have many years of experience as a licensed cosmetologist and must be qualified for a managerial position. It is very difficult to run an entire operation without responsible help to rely on. A good manager is critical to the life of a well-run salon. Last, but surely not least, the personality of the manager can make or break your beauty parlor. A pleasant, attractive, well-groomed, intelligent, warm, and efficient person can coordinate the entire business, making it a pleasant place for workers and patrons alike.

STATE REGULATION

Every state spells out in detail how a beauty salon should be set up and how it should function. In Washington, D.C., for example, the Cosmetological Act stipulates:

> It shall be unlawful for any person to practice cosmetology for pay in any place other than a registered beauty shop: Provided, That a registered operator may in an emergency furnish cosmetological treatments to persons in the permanent or temporary residences of such persons by appointment. Every beauty shop shall have a manager, who shall have immediate charge and supervision over the operators practicing cosmetology.

Licenses have to be obtained for cosmetology salons, too. The following describes how to proceed in the state of California in accordance with the regulations set forth by the California Department of Consumer Affairs. (Section numbers refer to specific code items.)

Cosmetological Establishments Defined

7380. A cosmetological establishment is any premises, building or part of a building, where is practiced any branch or any combination of branches of cosmetology, or the occupation of a cosmetologist, except the branch of manicuring as practiced in barber shops, licensed by the board and complying with the provisions of Sections 7381, 7382, 7383, and 7384 of this code and all sanitary regulations established by the board.

License Required

7381. Any person, firm, or corporation desiring to operate a cosmetological establishment shall make an application to the board for a certificate of registration and license, accompanied by the registration fee prescribed by this chapter. The applicant, if an individual, or each officer, director, and partner, if the applicant is other than an individual, shall not have committed acts or crimes which are grounds for denial of licensure under section 480. A certificate issued pursuant to this section shall authorize the operation of the establishment only at the location for which the certificate is issued. Operation of the establishment at any other location shall be unlawful unless a certificate for the new location has been obtained upon compliance with the provisions of this section applicable to the issuance of a certificate in the first instance.

Supervision of Establishments

7382. A cosmetological establishment shall, at all times, be in the charge of a licensed cosmetologist, except that if the operations within the establishment are limited to the practice of electrology, such establishment may, at all times be in the charge of a licensed electrologist, and if the operations within the establishment are limited to the practice of manicuring, such establishment may at all times, be in the charge of a licensed manicurist, and if the operations within the establishment are limited to the practice of a cosmetician, such establishment may, at all times, be in the charge of a licensed cosmetician.

Personnel Employed

7383. It is unlawful for any person to employ, or allow to be employed, or permit to work, in or about a cosmetological establishment any person who performs cosmetological services and is not duly registered or licensed by the board. Any person violating the provisions of this section is guilty of a misdemeanor.

OTHER REGULATIONS

After you have complied with the state codes, be careful to read all the local codes as well to be certain that you are not in violation. Careless misdemeanors can be costly.

Hairdressing and cosmetology rulings from the Department of State, Division of Licensing Services, Albany, New York, stipulates:

> All beauty parlors shall be maintained and operated in accordance with the provisions of the State Sanitary Code, except in the City of New York where the New York City Health Code shall apply, and all licensees or persons employed or engaged therein or in connection therewith shall comply with the provisions of such codes.

The New York City Health Code then proceeds to detail the amount, type, and correct usage of all equipment.

10.10 Water supply. An adequate supply of hot and cold water from a municipal or satisfactory private source shall be provided for service for customers, cleanliness of employees, and for washing floors, walls, ceiling and equipment.

10.11 Waste disposal. Waste water from all plumbing fixtures shall be discharged into municipal sewers where available. Otherwise suitable facilities shall be installed for the absorption of the wastes by the soil in the underground systems, so that no nuisance is created.

10.12 Plumbing fixtures. Plumbing fixtures shall be of impervious material and of a type which is readily cleanable. They shall be free from cracks and from parts which are not readily accessible for cleaning. They shall be of a type which does not constitute a hazard to a public water supply through back siphonage.

10.13 Floors. Floors shall be of such construction as to be easily cleaned and shall be kept clean and in good repair. If carpeting or similar material is used for floor covering, it shall be of a light color with a single loop pile of not more than one-quarter inch in height. Such floor covering shall be kept clean by vacuuming at least daily and shampooing at least annually and more frequently if the covering is not clean.

10.14 Lighting and ventilation. Lighting fixtures shall be in sufficient number and properly placed so as to provide adequate illumination. The shop shall be properly and adequately ventilated.

10.15 Cabinets. Cabinets shall be provided for storage of clean linen and towels. They shall have tight fitting doors that shall be kept closed to protect the linen and towels from dust and dirt.

10.17 Refuse. Covered containers for hair droppings, paper and other waste material shall be provided and maintained so that they are not offensive.

Though some of the stipulations are simple common sense, others are elaborately detailed requirements that you must follow to the letter when you open your salon. An unfavorable inspection could prevent you from opening if you are not within the code.

FINDING A LOCATION

After you have carefully established what constitutes a cosmetology business, you will want to familiarize yourself with the location and building floor plan you have chosen for your beauty salon. The first thing to consider is finding a good location where you will not be in direct competition with another beauty salon. Even with a large following you will need to have favorable conditions to succeed in your own business. Next you should ask if the place is large enough for expansion, or whether you will have to consider moving in a few years. Will it be inconvenient to your clientele if you do move after you are once established? Could you possibly afford to open another salon to accommodate a prosperous business? Will this be a convenient place for your staff to reach? You cannot possibly foresee all the "ifs." But a little foresight could help you decide on the location of your place of business.

When you invest in equipment for your salon, be certain that it is the best quality, because repairs of inferior plumbing and other equipment will cost many times more than if you had paid for good equipment at the beginning.

HIRING A STAFF AND GETTING STARTED

Once the final decision to own your own salon has started to become a reality, you will have to hire a congenial staff with professional knowledge and assets that will attract customers to your salon. Word-of-mouth is always the best advertisement, so you will want to employ hairstylists with good followings who will expand your business. It will be critical to your new salon to have some established clientele. Starting from the beginning and building a clientele is possible, but if prospective patrons see that you are busy with at least a few customers, their confidence will bring them to you more quickly.

You will have to decide the cost of your services, another "make-or-break" factor. Your operators deserve to be paid commensurate with their ability, so familiarize yourself with the area where you will have your salon and get a sense of the income of the potential clientele.

You will have to use common sense and a lot of intuition to start out. Your prices will rise, as with all businesses, but you will have to encourage new patrons, give good services, keep your prices within reason, and realize profits to continue. It will take a clever balance of good salesmanship and good will to keep you afloat.

Most of your operators will be bringing patrons along with them from their last place of employment, so the practice of paying the operator a percentage will be a workable arrangement for both of you. The percentage must be large enough to induce the operator to continue to work for you and also to want to build up her or his following. Tips are a sizable income course, and most operators realize as much as another thirty to thirty-five percent of their salary in tips.

Hiring an Accountant

Bookkeeping is another very important part of your beauty salon. It is vital to the life of your investment to have accurate bookkeeping. You may have a talent for this area, and in a very small place, you could keep track of all expenditures, income, inventory, repairs, and fees. As your business grows, it is the profit and loss statistics that will guide you in hiring a qualified accountant. Accountants do the job most efficiently and save you money in the long run. A good accountant points out all the areas where you can improve your income, increase your insurance if necessary, cut back on excess personnel, and generally make things orderly. An accountant will be an invaluable aid to you not only in advising you before you purchase a salon, but also in the annual bookkeeping. He or she will be able to tell you how to control your expenses and how to realize greater profits. You will also have to deal with business taxes. Your accountant will seem like an expense until you see how difficult it is to figure all the expenditures on your own. Many hours must be spent with the financial juggling of even the smallest business. Tax laws change annually, and the accountant can keep you abreast of all the critical matters without endless hours of research on your part.

Taking Out Insurance

Insurance is another expenditure involved in owning your own place of business. Especially in the cosmetology field, malpractice insurance is a must. Even the most careful operator is human and capable of injuring a customer. A permanent solution could be left on too long, or even after testing, a patron could have a violent allergic reaction. If a patron sues for negligence and wins, you as the salon owner could lose everything that you have worked so hard to build up. Malpractice insurance can protect you, and it is foolhardy not to have it.

Fire insurance is also essential. If the amount of your total investment in your equipment alone were lost, could you afford to replace it? Fire insurance would cover the interior and the exterior of your shop. This kind of insurance should be brought up to date annually, as inflation causes the replacement prices to be higher than the original investment.

Insurance should also cover possible burglary. A few years ago, it would have been extremely uncommon to have equipment stolen from a place like a beauty salon. Now it is wise to cover all equipment, retail stock, and beauty supplies with this type of insurance. The cost of replacing them could mean the difference between closing your business or buying new equipment and starting again.

Liability insurance on the actual premises is another type of insurance that you will have to maintain. If a patron or an employee is injured in your salon, a serious lawsuit could ensue. Depending on the outcome of the damages awarded, a suit could not only put you out of business but into personal debt as well. Accidents can and do happen, and you should be prepared by taking out this kind of insurance.

Some states require that you carry worker's compensation insurance. On-the-job injuries or work-related illness could cause the employee to miss work and lose pay. Worker's compensation pays the employee until he or she can return to work. If your state requires this type of insurance and you are negligent in carrying it, a lawsuit could conceivably put you out of business. Check your state's rulings. Even if your state does not require it, you may find yourself being sued for such a case. Worker's compensation insurance could save you financially.

THE KEY TO SUCCESS

Being nice to your customers is only common sense if you want their business. And happy patrons tell their friends how happy they are with your services. But there is something more than just exterior politeness. You must be honest, fair, loyal, and respectful, not only to the paying clientele but to all your employees as well. Businesslike and considerate methods should keep your salon working at its optimum. If the atmosphere is pleasant and congenial, everyone who comes in touch with your salon will be comfortable and want to return. Your business needs this sort of professionalism to be a lasting success.

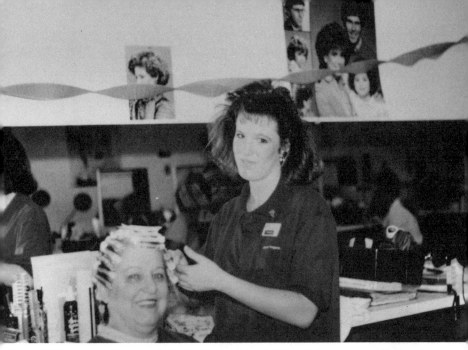

Top: State regulations require beauty schools to provide their students with the equipment they need to practice their skills. (Capri School of Beauty Culture, Inc. photo) *Bottom*: A cosmetology instructor demonstrates proper manicuring techniques. (Pittsburgh Beauty Academy photo)

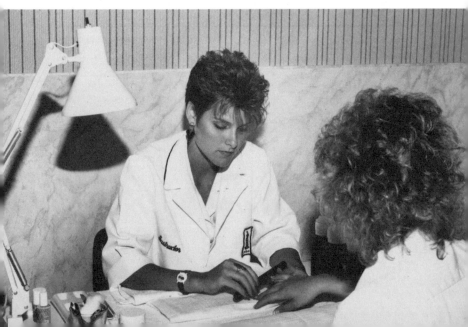

CHAPTER 12

OWNING AND MANAGING
A BEAUTY SCHOOL

Owning a beauty school can be a very large and profitable business. Almost 10,000 students graduated from beauty schools in California alone during the 1986 school year. Tuition costs run from $1500 to $2000 per student depending on the area and the type of beauty school.

SCHOOLS OF COSMETOLOGY AND
SCHOOLS OF ELECTROLOGY REGULATIONS

Specific regulations spell out every detail set down in state codes. The following regulations are from the Cosmetology Act issued by the California Board of Cosmetology.

Application to Conduct School of Cosmetology

910. (a) An application for a license to conduct a school of cosmetology or school of electrology shall be submitted on an application form prescribed and provided by the board, accompanied by such evidence, statements or documents as therein required, and filed with the board at its office in Sacramento.

(b) An inspector of the board shall make a preliminary inspection of the proposed school premises and shall submit a report to the board.

(c) A second inspection of the proposed school premises shall be made by an inspector after the minimum equipment has been installed therein, and a report of such inspection shall be made to the board before a school license is issued.

Minimum Space for Schools of Cosmetology

911. (a) The minimum ceiling height of the practice and classroom areas of school premises shall be sufficient to insure adequate air, light, and ventilation. A minimum ceiling height of nine feet shall be presumed to be adequate for such purposes.

(b) The minimum floor space in any school of cosmetology premises shall be 3000 square feet, not less than 2000 square feet of which shall be provided for the working, practice, and classroom areas.

(c) When the average daily attendance for either day school or night school in a school of cosmetology exceeds fifty students for a period of three months, additional floor space shall be provided sufficient for the proper instruction and training of such additional students.

Equipment for Schools of Cosmetology

912. (a) The minimum equipment for a school of cosmetology shall be as follows:

1. Sufficient electrical equipment and dermal lights for giving instruction in skin care and electrical facials. Equipment shall be capable of producing galvanic, faradic, and sinusoidal currents. Said electrical equipment and lights shall be required effective October 1, 1980.

2. Ten mannequins, with full head of hair

3. One time clock

4. Five shampoo bowls
   (When the average daily attendance exceeds fifty students, additional shampoo bowls shall be added at the ratio of one for each twenty-five students in average daily attendance in excess of fifty.)

5. Twelve dryers
   (When the average daily attendance exceeds fifty students, additional dryers shall be added at the ratio of one for each ten students in average daily attendance in excess of fifty.)

6. Four facial chairs or facial couches
   (When the average daily attendance exceeds fifty students, additional facial chairs or facial couches shall be added at the ratio of one for each twenty-five students in average daily attendance in excess of fifty.)

7. Six manicure stations
   (When the average daily attendance exceeds fifty students, additional manicure tables shall be added at the ratio of one for each ten students in average daily attendance in excess of fifty.)

8. One electrical cap
   (When the average daily attendance exceeds fifty students, additional electrical caps shall be added at the ratio of one for each twenty-five students in average daily attendance in excess of fifty.)

9. Thermal hair straighteners, including:
   one electric comb
   three nonelectric combs
   one stove for nonelectric combs
   one electric curling iron
   three nonelectric curling irons (at least two sizes)
   one stove for nonelectric curling irons

   (b) The minimum equipment for a school of cosmetology conducting a course in electrology shall also include the following:

1. Either one high frequency generator (thermolysis) machine plus one galvanic generator (electrolysis) machine or one combination thermolysis/electrolysis machine capable of furnishing training in both thermolysis and electrolysis

2. Four needles of various sizes ranging from 0.003 to 0.008 of an inch

3. One dispersive or inactive electrode with connections to the machine, such as wet pad, metal rod, or water jar, necessary for electrology treatments only

4. One lamp and bulb (if bulb is of the exposed type, at least 60-watt strength is required)

5. One stool, adjustable in height

6. One table or chair for patrons

7. One utility stand for set-up

8. One towel cabinet

9. Six covered containers for lotions, soaps, sterilizing agents, and cotton

10. One container for immersing needles for sterilization purposes

11. One container for immersing eye pads in solution

12. One fine-pointed epilation forceps
    (When the average daily attendance in a course of electrology or thermology exceeds three students for a two-month period, one additional complete set of equipment shall be added for each three students in average daily attendance in excess of three.)

(c) The minimum equipment for a school of cosmetology conducting a course in wig styling shall also include the following:

Five blocks in various sizes from nineteen to twenty-three inches with holders.

(When the average daily attendance for student enrolled in a wig styling course exceeds five, additional blocks with holders shall be added at the ratio of one for each additional student.)

(d) Each school shall designate a specific area in which practical training in facials shall be conducted. Such area shall be of sufficient size to accommodate the four facial chairs or couches required by subdivision (a) of this section, and all of such chairs and couches shall remain in the area designated as the facial area at all times during which the school is conducting instruction and training. No chair shall be used as a facial chair unless it is equipped with a headrest and footrest which makes it suitable for the purpose.

Equipment for Schools Conducting a Course in Electrology

912.1 The minimum equipment for a school of electrology and schools of cosmetology conducting a course in electrology shall consist of:

(a) Current Generators:

Either one high frequency generator (thermolysis) and one galvanic generator (electrolysis) machine, or one high frequency generator (thermolysis) and one blend machine capable of producing both the high frequency and galvanic current.

(One additional current generator of those listed above shall be required when the average daily attendance exceeds each multiple of three students.)

(b) The equipment to be used with each required generator shall include:

1. One dozen needles including all graduations from 0.002 to 0.006

2. Lamp and bulb

3. Stool adjustable in height

4. Table or chair for patron

5. Utility stand

6. Sufficient number of covered containers for lotions, soaps, sterilizing agents, contaminated instruments, and cotton

7. Two fine-pointed epilation forceps

(c) Equipment for sterilizing electrolysis needles and tweezers by all of the methods prescribed in Section 981

(d) A time clock

Student's Books and Instruments

912.2. The term *books* shall be limited to texts and manuals dealing with the art of cosmetology or any of its branches and the term *instruments* shall be limited to hand tools and implements, operated by hand whenever in use. The board may determine whether any book or instrument is reasonably necessary to a student's instruction.

The size of the building required by the state will obviously be your first consideration when buying space for a cosmetology school. The state dictates what dimensions are a must. In large cities rental costs could be very expensive. The equipment is also stipulated, and certain numbers of employees will be set by those same boards. All possible financial costs should be weighed carefully, and you should consult with advisors on the best way to start your own business. Rental, buying, or even taking over someone else's established beauty school can all be serious decisions. Mortgages and down payments may be something that you are already familiar with, but if this is your first business, you will want all of the latest advice for taxes and deductions and insurance.

REGULATIONS IN CALIFORNIA

Not all states are as specific as California when it comes to details of cosmetology laws. California's definitions are more precise than many other states', and for that reason, it provides a good example.

Schools

7390. Schools of cosmetology and schools of electrology shall be conducted as provided in this article.

License Required

7391. Any person, firm, or corporation desiring to conduct a school of cosmetology or a school of electrology shall make an application to the board for a certificate of registration of license. The application shall be accompanied by the school application fee and the school inspection fee prescribed in this chapter.

If the board determines after completion of the inspections required by this chapter that the applicant is entitled to the issuance of a license sought, it shall issue such license upon the payment of the annual registration fee prescribed by this chapter, prorates in accordance with the number of months remaining in the license years, commencing with and including the month in which the license is issued.

Renewal of School Licenses

7438. Certificates of registration for schools of cosmetology and schools of electrology expire on September 30th of each year. An application for renewal of a certificate shall be filed with the board during the month of August or September, accompanied by the annual registration fee prescribed by this chapter. Thereupon the board shall renew the certificate for the ensuing year.

A certificate which has expired for failure of the registrant to renew within the time fixed by this section may for a period of one year thereafter be renewed upon the filing of an application in such form as the board may require and upon payment of the annual registration fee and the delinquency fee provided by this chapter. After one year from the date of its expiration, a certificate may not be renewed, and the school may again become entitled to a certificate only upon compliance with all of the provisions of this chapter relating to the original issuance of a certificate.

Fees for Schools

7445. The amount of the fees required by this chapter relating to licenses to conduct schools of cosmetology or electrology shall be set by the board at not more than the amounts shown in the following schedule:

(a) The application fee for a school of cosmetology or a school of electrology shall be not more than $90.

(b) The inspection fee for a school of cosmetology or a school of electrology shall be not more than $90.

(c) The annual registration fee for a school of cosmetology or a school of electrology shall be not more than $225.

(d) The delinquency fee is $25.

School License

7392. The certificate of registration and license authorizes the school of cosmetology or the school of electrology holding it to transact operations in this state only on the premises approved by the board during the year or fraction thereof for which it is issued, subject to the rules and regulations of the board. In the event the holder of the school of cosmetology or school of electrology license proposes to conduct a part of his [or her] school activity on premises other than those heretofore licensed by the board, then such licensee shall obtain an additional license for the newly proposed premises as a school of electrology or a school of cosmetology. Nothing in this article shall be construed as authorization or permission to conduct a school of cosmetology or a school of electrology without a valid, existing, and unexpired certificate of registration covering the premises where such school is conducted.

Supervision of Schools

7392.2. Every school of cosmetology shall, at all times, be in the charge of and under the immediate supervision of a licensed cosmetology instructor, who has had at least a total of two years of continuous teaching experience in all branches of cosmetology, except electrology, in a licensed school in this state, after being duly licensed as an instructor under this chapter. Any person who within the five-year period immediately prior to September 17, 1965, has been registered with the board as a supervising instructor, shall be deemed to have the teaching experience required by this section.

Every person who instructs students in a school of cosmetology shall hold a valid California cosmetology instructor license.

All instructors shall be continuously engaged in teaching students in theoretical or practical work. Except when instructing a student and the student is doing the manual work, no instructor may practice upon a patron and any instructor who does so is subject to disciplinary action by the board.

School License Qualifications

7393. Before any school of cosmetology license shall be finally granted, a second inspection shall be made after the equipment has been installed and before the school is permitted to begin operation.

No applicant shall be granted a license to operate a school of cosmetology unless, in the opinion of the board, sufficient equipment has been installed for the requirements of enrolling a minimum of twenty-five bona fide students. No applicant shall be granted a license to operate a school of cosmetology or electrology unless the proposed school has such floor space and equipment as the board may prescribe by regulation as being reasonably necessary to provide a proper place for instruction and training.

No school of cosmetology shall be licensed until the board has had ample opportunity to verify sworn statements as to the actual ownership. If false statements are submitted to the board in connection with such application, this in itself shall constitute sufficient grounds for the refusal to grant any application hereunder, or if an application is granted and thereafter the board discovers that false statements were made in connection therewith, this shall constitute sufficient grounds for the cancellation of such school of cosmetology license even though it is detected after a license has been issued.

The board may deny a school of cosmetology license to any applicant who fails to present satisfactory evidence of personal integrity and moral responsibility, and in the event that such application is a corporation, this requirement shall apply to all the officers of such corporation. No school of cosmetology license, however, shall be issued until the real owner files with the department a statement definitely designating who is authorized to accept service of notice from the board and to transact all business negotiations in behalf of such school, including answers to citations for hearing and compliance with rulings issued by the board.

Change in Officers

7393.1 A corporation which holds a cosmetology school license shall notify the board in writing within fifteen days after a person becomes an officer of the corporation who was not an officer at the time the license was issued to the corporation. If, after proceedings conducted in accordance with the provisions of Chapter 5 (commencing with Section 11500) of Part I of Division 3 of Title 2 of the Government Code, to which the corporation shall be made a party, the board determines that any fact or condition exists as to the new officer which would be grounds for the suspension or revocation of a license under this chapter, it may order the corporation to remove the officer. Failure of the corporation to comply with such order within fifteen days after the order is served upon it shall result in the automatic suspension of its license until the officer is removed.

Student Enrollment

7393.3 (a) No applicant shall be granted a license to operate a school of cosmetology unless he [or she] first presents to the board evidence that at least twenty-five persons are enrolled as bona fide, full-time students for a course of training of the minimum number of hours required by this chapter for licensing as a cosmetologist.

(b) For purposes of this section, a person enrolled as a bona fide, full-time student is a person who has been entered on the roll of a proposed school of cosmetology which has met the requirements prescribed by the board, and who verifies that he [or she] will become a *bona fide* student by having committed himself [or herself] by contract to attend a full course in cosmetology.

(c) No contract referred to in subdivision (b) shall bind the prospective student if the proposed school of cosmetology does not begin instruction within ninety days after the contract is entered into.

(d) Such students shall not have been enrolled in a school of cosmetology within one year immediately preceding the date of application for enrollment.

(e) This section shall not apply to a transfer of an existing school license from premises, or a transfer of an existing school to a new owner or ownership.

School Advertising

7393.5 No school of cosmetology shall advertise services to the public through any medium, including radio, unless such services are expressly designated as student work.

School Equipment

7395. Every school shall possess sufficient apparatus and equipment necessary for the ready and full teaching of all subjects or practices of cosmetology.

School Staff

7396. Every school of cosmetology shall maintain licensed instructors competent to impart instruction in all branches or practices of cosmetology.

Financial Ability

7396.6 No applicant shall be granted a license to operate a school of cosmetology or a school of electrology unless he [or she] shall submit evidence satisfactory to the board of his [or her] financial ability to provide the facilities and equipment required by the board regulation and to maintain the operation of the proposed school for a period of one year.

Attendance

7397. Every school shall keep a daily record of the attendance of each student and the time devoted by each student to the various practices or branches of cosmetology and electrology. It shall establish grades and hold examinations before issuing diplomas.

No student shall be required or permitted to attend more than eight hours of instruction or practice, or any combination thereof,

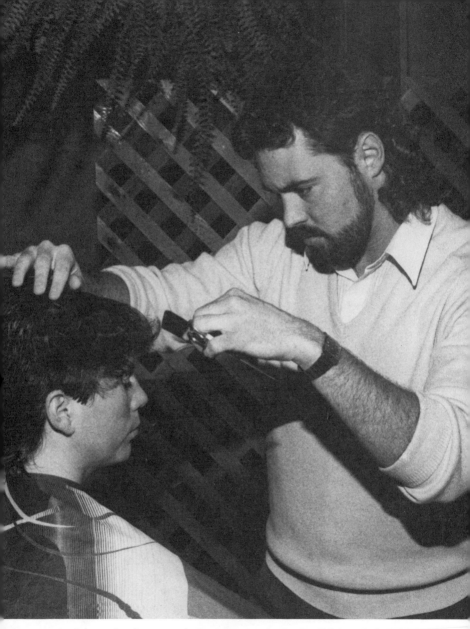

Job openings for cosmetologists are expected to be plentiful through the year 2000. (Pittsburgh Beauty Academy photo)

in any one day, except that a student may be permitted to complete a service in process, but not to exceed thirty consecutive minutes.

School Bond

7398. Every school shall post with the board a good and sufficient surety bond executed by the applicant as principal and by a surety company as surety in the amount of $5,000.

The bond shall be in the form approved by the board and shall be conditioned upon compliance with the provisions of this chapter and upon faithful compliance with the terms and conditions of any and all contracts, verbal or written made by the school to furnish instruction to any person. The bond shall be to the State of California in favor of every person who pays or deposits any money with the school as payment for any instruction. Every bond shall continue in force and effect until notice of termination is given by registered mail to the board and every bond shall set forth this fact.

Any person claiming to be injured or damaged by any act of the school may maintain an action on the bond against the school and the surety named therein, or either of them, for refund of tuition paid and any judgment against the principal or surety in any such action shall include the costs thereof and those incident to the bringing of the action, including a reasonable attorney fee. The aggregate liability of the surety to all such persons shall not, however, exceed the sum of the bond.

Tuition

7398.5 Every school shall fix its tuition at such an amount as will enable it to furnish without further charge to the student all cosmetics, materials and supplies used on the public and in classes. This does not include books and instruments.

Fees for Schools

7445. The amount of the fees required by this chapter relating to licenses to conduct schools of cosmetology or electrology shall be set by the board at not more than the amounts shown in the following schedule:

(a) The application fee for a school of cosmetology or a school of electrology shall be not more than $90.

(b) The inspection fee for a school of cosmetology or a school of electrology shall be not more than $90.

(c) The annual registration fee for a school of cosmetology or a school of electrology shall be not more than $225.

(d) The delinquency fee is $25.

All states have similar stipulations for owning a school of cosmetology, though they do not have as many restrictions, and they are usually not as well defined as these. The operation of a school of this nature takes serious endeavor on the part of the owner or owners. The success of the school depends on the owner's ability to meet all the financial needs, the legal prerequisites, and the needs of the staff and students. Location and student enrollment obviously dictate income potential.

There are strict health regulations that govern the physical plant as to plumbing, floor coverings, windows (number of and coverings for), fire code compliance, number and sanitation of toilets, and provisions for pest control. Cleanliness and sanitation are paramount in a beauty school due to the nature of its services.

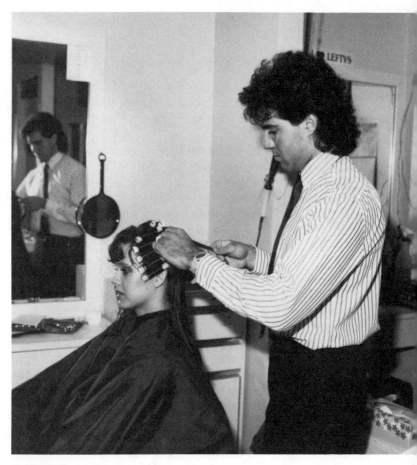

(Pittsburgh Beauty Academy photo)

CHAPTER 13

MANAGING THE SALON

The position of the managing cosmetologist (manager-operator) is often considered the intermediate post between doing cosmetological work and owning a salon. Each state dictates prerequisites, such as the amount of schooling needed, years of cosmetology experience, and manager-operator licensing. A manager-cosmetologist earns an annual income of about $22,000 in larger cities. The actual number of patrons whom a cosmetologist brings to the salon for weekly services has a great effect on his or her salary level.

Certain managerial positions are geared toward promotion, while others are strictly business coordination. The emphasis depends on the size of the salon and the salary arrangement.

One New York City department store manager considers his main responsibility as business. He does not dress hair, nor does he have to be licensed by the state of New York. He is a man of responsibility, charm, and efficiency. His work consists of hiring, firing, maintaining inventory, overseeing the bookkeeping, and seeing to schedules for daily work and holidays for all employees. He is paid a percentage of the salon's profits and feels that this arrangement gives him more incentive to work, as his income is not limited.

The manager-operator must be licensed as a cosmetologist by the state in which he or she works. The manager-operator is permitted to touch the patron and do hairstyles, unlike the manager who is not a cosmetologist. States require varying levels of experience as a licensed operator before application can be made for the manager-operator license. Some states will permit operators to apply for that particular license as soon as they have started to work in a salon.

The advantage of having been an operator prior to taking a managerial position is that being familiar with all aspects of the cosmetology business is helpful in numerous ways. You may be permitted to suggest improvements, such as the introduction of new equipment or even a cosmetic line bearing your salon's signature. All of these factors directly influence your income.

A MANAGER'S RESPONSIBILITIES

As a manager-cosmetologist, you would be directly responsible for the entire coordination and running of the business. Linens have to be rented and laundered, supplies have to be kept in stock, and equipment has to be kept up-to-date and in working order.

It would be your obligation to keep abreast of regulations, and you would have to read new codes annually. The decor of the salon may be one of your responsibilities. You must learn to balance economy with attractive surroundings. There are many kinds of managerial positions, so you will definitely want to have all of your areas of authority spelled out clearly.

Avoid being in a position where more and more work is expected of you without salary adjustments. You will be managing the largest portion of the business end of the salon. With the exception of paying rent or mortgage payments and directing funds for business expenses, you could conceivably be running the entire salon. You may even be managing the money for the owners. Coordinating the entire operation and suffering the headaches that accompany that amount of responsibility makes the manager's position the highest paid of the salon employees.

The wage scale varies from state to state, salon to salon. Anything above minimum wage, and often well above $450 a week can be expected in larger cities. The location of the salon will definitely have an influence on your salary. If the customers are paying above average for services, the salary for a manager would be comparable. In a small local salon, the responsibilities may be of greater variety, but the pay would obviously have to be in line with the income of the shop.

Managers are normally expected to work the longest hours as well. A manager has to oversee the entire workings of the salon and must be aware of problems before they become too difficult to handle.

The hiring of personnel is very important. Keeping a happy, congenial group must always be paramount in the manager's mind. One unpleasant employee, no matter how talented, can cause miserable working conditions for everyone in the salon.

The quality of the workmanship is what will make or break your salon's future. If you do have skilled hairstylists, word-of-mouth will interest others, and your clientele will increase.

One of the jobs of the manager is unfortunately policing. He or she has to make certain that all licenses are current for every operator, the salon, and of course for him or herself if the state requires a manager's license.

Enforcement of all sanitary rules is also one of a manager's responsibilities. If your salon suffered a lawsuit because one of your operators was negligent, your employer, the salon owner, would certainly be looking for a new manager. So to protect yourself and everyone else, policy should be clearly stated at the beginning, and everyone will know what is expected of him or her and how he or she is to conduct him or herself under your management. In case of a critical problem, management will have to be the arbitrator, and short of a lawsuit, your wisdom will have to prevail. Experience is usually a great help when these crises arise, but there will always be a "first," and how you handle the situation will be noted by your underlings as well as your boss.

Diplomat, overseer, personnel coordinator, inventory controller, host, record and schedule keeper—these are the responsibilities of the manager.

The number of positions open to managers are few. Many salon owners prefer to manage their own salon. If you are interested in management, you may do well to consult trade periodicals and a large city newspaper's want ads.

CHAPTER 14

COMPETITION STYLISTS

There are many reasons you might want to enter hairdressers' competitions. If you are planning on making a career in hairstyling, you really should consider applying to as many competitions as possible. There are numerous benefits. You will meet many people in your chosen field, and you will be able to observe first-hand the best cosmetologists. Exposure to many clever hairdressers is a tremendous learning experience.

You have the advantage of being able to enter competitions as early as your days in beauty school. The confidence that you can gain in competition is worth every penny of your entrance fees. Competitions are also very exciting. Prizes range from trophies to cash, and many contacts are made during these shows that can lead to recognition in the cosmetology world. The press covers all the proceedings, and many fine cosmetologists have gained a following through competition.

COMPETITIONS

Hair competition for a cosmetology student would most likely consist of a daytime haircut, style, or other already familiar technique. The experience of competing gives the student a better idea of accuracy, speed, and the correct method of attaining an end result at someone's request. When the pressure is on, some students function at their best. Others simply cannot cope with all the confusion and noise and are better off in the slower pace of school. This does not mean that if you have trouble at your first competition you should not consider entering competitions in the future, after you have gained experience and confidence.

There are also competitions for students of barbering schools who must quickly and skillfully perform a man's cut and present their model with a final polished look. The haircut itself may be judged separately.

Competitions are sponsored by a variety of groups. The most common sponsor is the larger manufacturer of products like hairdressings or makeup, publishers of cosmetology magazines, and affiliations of cosmetologists. Competitions occur frequently.

Areas of Competition

The professional has many different choices of areas in which to compete. One specialty for competition is permanent waving. There are many ways in which hair can be set and styled to achieve a particular look. Piggybacking is one method currently used to set permanents. The choice of wrapping method makes a remarkable difference. The corkscrew method of curling the hair on the rod is a recent technique. You could perm only the base of the hair, or only the ends of the hair, or the entire length of the hair. All of these techniques give a wide variety of hairstyles and enable you to achieve innovative results.

Time allotment is critical, so have everything organized in your mind ahead of time. Judges are usually a panel of several authorities in the field. You will be told the theme or silhouette to be achieved, and whether it is to be a daytime or evening hairstyle. Be certain that you and your model are available at the prescribed hour, as latecomers are turned away, and your entrance fee probably will not be refunded.

Some possible competitions could be creative coloring, creative or "open" hairstyling (the contestant can create any style or type of hair design such as disco, high fashion, day, or evening), men's styling competition by a cosmetologist (no barbers permitted to enter), creative cutting, or dual competition, wherein one male and one female model are styled by the same contestant to show the operator's ability to "cross over." (Formerly, *unisex* was the term used to describe hairstyling for both men and women.) There are competitions for permanent waving, and even contests wherein the cosmetologist creates an entire fashion look. The contestant coordinates hair, makeup, and even clothing to present a total look.

REASONS FOR COMPETING

Competitions are held at the lower levels for the operator to gain experience, to develop a better time record for setting and comb-outs, and to acquire a reputation. Winning competitions is a good way to become recognized and to increase clientele. Sometimes the prize is money, a trophy, or a plaque engraved with recognition of award or merit. Many operators and beauty salon owners announce their most prestigious awards in their advertisements and on business cards.

One of the best reasons to enter competition is just for fun. It is an opportunity for creativity and innovation. When you work in a salon, you must consider the wishes of the client. Not so at competitions! Restrictions are set down prior to entering, and you can enter the competition of your choice as long as you are qualified. You supply your own model and work with him or her exclusively. The rules will dictate to the letter what colors are acceptable and how they may be used, what type of rollers or clips you may use and even how you are to dry hair. Any electric devices you will need have to be stated prior to the onset of the competition, and you will be advised as to available outlets and wattage.

Competitions are a chance for you to learn by observing. The best in the field are represented at competitions, and you can watch genuine talent. By the time that the advanced and very highly skilled cosmetologists are competing, the prizes are more prestigious. International teams enter against other famous international teams in olympic hairstyling competitions. As you might have guessed, these contests are quite spectacular for hair fashion as well as for the latest in clothing. Designer clothes and hairstyles blend in this level of competition, and the model is presented with a complete look. Even if a model is dressed in the most glamorous gown, the effect is ruined if her hair is not styled properly. So this is where the hairstylist can really shine. A beautiful and well-thought-out hair creation (one that truly benefits the model and the mood) can make the whole presentation.

Hair competition can keep you well abreast of current styles. For a competition, no dated hair style is requested or permitted. There are many benefits to be gained from entering contests: education, experience, a wider scope of the field of cosmetology (particularly how it fits into the beauty world), confidence in yourself and in your chosen craft, recognition for personal ability and talents as well as publicity and status for the salon that you own or where you are currently employed, and last, but not least, your awards in trophy or cash prizes.

There are endless competitions at all levels of experience and talent. You may want to compete alone or as a team member from your salon. You may some day be talented and famous enough to compete on the international level with years of solid experience behind you and recognition throughout the entire cosmetology world. The best part of entering competition styling is that it is wide open to students, professionals, small-town salon operators and big-city, high fashion stylists, males, and females. You will never know what you could be winning unless you compete!

CHAPTER 15

PLATFORM STYLISTS

A platform stylist is a polished artist who has become established in the world of creative cosmetology or trendsetting. These stylists are recognized for their outstanding ability in hairstyling and are employed by salons to teach their operators the latest looks. Product manufacturers also employ platform stylists to demonstrate their products and equipment. These specialists draw hourly wages from $50 to $100 depending upon the area, the size of the audience, and the product.

THE ROLE OF THE PLATFORM STYLIST

Platform stylists are really teachers with much more savvy and awareness of hair trends—both immediate and future—than the average operator. Most teachers and operators are engrossed in the daily routine of styling patrons' hair. Keeping up-to-date is a critical problem for all hairstylists. Unless a style is acceptably current, few patrons will want to wear it. Even the standby short permed hairstyle for the elderly patron has become softer and more natural looking. So not only must operators know present hairstyles, but a good operator must have a constant awareness of the latest trend and even future trends. Younger people in particular are extremely demanding in their desire to wear the latest trend or even be pacesetters. There are many salons whose managers hire platform stylists regularly to enlighten the entire staff.

It would be extremely costly and, in a small salon, truly impossible for all the cosmetologists to return to school as often as hair fashions change. With a platform stylist visiting and teaching in the beauty salon, every person benefits. The operators do not have to lose even a day's work since the platform stylist is usually scheduled to give lectures and demonstrations during the hours immediately before or directly after the salon's business hours. By being in the work environment, the operator can more easily visualize how and with what equipment new hairstyles will be created. Busier salons can afford to have a few operators ask the platform stylist questions during lengthier sessions as other operators continue to work. Some instructors do platform stylist work as well as beauty school instruction on an advanced level. There are many ways in the beauty industry to combine the various aspects of the cosmetology trade, just as long as you are practicing in a state that does not require more education than you have or a different license from the one that you hold.

There has been some discussion about requiring licensed cosmetologists to refresh themselves annually with continuing education courses. New laws and regulations are about to appear in several states.

The platform stylist teaches only techniques, and continuing education courses are geared to business and management.

BECOMING A PLATFORM STYLIST

The platform stylist can expect to earn about $400 for four to eight hours of work. Some very famous platform stylists earn a thousand dollars a day for their instruction. Supply houses, cosmetic firms, and sometimes affiliates sponsor platform stylists. A normal schedule for a well-qualified platform stylist might be giving lectures and instruction only twice a month. It is not an everyday job, and most of these "teachers" work in managerial or operator positions in salons. Some platform stylists take their lecture, instruction, slides, and models from place to place. But their schedule is almost never full time.

The platform stylist's work necessitates both having up-to-the-second information on the "in" hairstyle and knowing how to create it. The former is obviously easier to come by. Some of the complexities of accomplishing a particular look are really very trying. It takes patience and an adaptable mind to be able to master one technique after another. Some extremely complex styles demand hours of fine hair coloring and then several more hours of hair wrapping to achieve the desired outcome. Often, shortly after gaining proficiency in a certain technique, that technique is on its way out. Then you have to struggle to grasp the new technique before you lose customers who desire the new hairstyle.

Hairdressing is very much a part of the fashion world and change is constant. It is a challenge to some operators, and an impossibility for others, to learn the new techniques necessary to create the latest trend. Somehow it has always been the innovators in the hairdressing world, like those in the fashion world of clothing, who have caught the attention of the fashion-conscious and held it over the years. Very avant-garde hairstyles, such as the asymmetricals a few years ago, are just what the fashion people love. Hairstylists spark their imaginations and give them a creating force or impetus. Hairstylists must have constant input; the fashion world never stands still. The platform stylist is therefore very necessary. And with a reasonable amount of ambition and perseverance it can be a very rewarding job.

Another advantage of working as a platform stylist is the potential for travel. But extensive travel may not be necessary. If you want to stay in a general vicinity, taking your newly learned knowledge to an area with a smaller radius, you could conceivably stay within several counties or states. Or you could find yourself lecturing in other countries. As fashion travels, so must hairstyle techniques. We in the United States often adapt French or English hair fashions. This offers a great opportunity for the platform stylist to learn the method and transport it.

FINDING A JOB

A platform stylist finds work through first establishing him or herself as a competition stylist. The demand for his or her work could eventually lead to actual platform work when available.

In certain states, a platform license is required. This license is applied for only once and lasts as long as the stylist maintains an active cosmetology license.

Work as a platform stylist can be acquired through hiring a booking agent. Some stylists simply free-lance if their contacts are already established through a hairdressing affiliate.

CHAPTER 16

EMPLOYMENT OUTLOOK FOR COSMETOLOGISTS

JOB OPPORTUNITIES

The United States Department of Labor's 1988-89 edition of the *Occupational Outlook Handbook* offers the following projections for opportunities in cosmetology:

> Job openings for cosmetologists are expected to be plentiful through the year 2000. Most openings will result from the need to replace the large number of workers who leave the occupation each year—primarily to devote full time to household responsibilities. Employment of cosmetologists is expected to grow about as fast as the average for all occupations through the year 2000 in response to population growth, particularly among middle-aged persons, who are the primary users of cosmetology services, and the rising number of working women. Hairstyling for men also contributes to the demand for cosmetologists because many men go to full-service shops or cosmetology salons for styling services. Opportunities for part-time work should continue to be very good.

In 1986, there were about 595,000 cosmetologists employed in the United States. They worked in beauty salons, unisex shops, department stores, hospitals, and hotels. In 1960, statistics show that only 300,000 persons were employed cosmetologists. At that time, the projected growth was only thousands. In fact, the figure very nearly doubled. It is obvious that this particular field is expanding greatly, and if it continues at the indicated pace, there will be many jobs available through the 1990s.

In California alone, there are approximately 50,000 employed cosmetologists, and the projected job openings in that state are 4,550 per year. Nearly 10,000 cosmetology students graduate every year from California beauty schools. Though this situation has existed for several years, it does not seem to have affected the demand for cosmetologists in California, according to the *California Occupational Guide.*

Even if the projections are somewhat contradictory, the overall picture for the future of cosmetology is an exceptionally bright one. There are many people who complete cosmetology schooling, take the state boards, become licensed operators, and then do not seek full-time employment. The statistics only tell us how many persons hold cosmetology licenses and do not go into detail as to how often, or even if, many of these operators join in the work force. There will always be openings for qualified hairstylists. The demand is continuing and growing. All the cosmetology services need to be filled to capacity, and there are jobs continuously becoming available.

SALARIES

Average earnings for a cosmetologist who is just starting out amount to between $12,000 and $13,000 per year. The projected increase is about $20,000 as soon as he or she has an established clientele. Remember that this is an average figure, and that there are cities where the salary could be much higher and less-populated areas where it could be lower. Tips are notably larger in the bigger cities and easily could amount to one-third of the wage.

Salaries and commissions normally are negotiated before an operator accepts a position with a salon. Much depends upon the experience and the following that the operator is bringing into the salon. If a large following will accompany the operator, it is not in his or her best interest to settle for a straight salary. Obviously the clientele will continue to increase, and the operator should benefit as well as the salon owner.

Commission arrangements are normally forty to fifty percent of the total for the operator. Only if an operator had no following and was just starting out would he or she consider a minimum guaranteed salary. Specialists and stylists with experience earned salaries around $15,000 a year in the mid- and late 1970s. Those same operators are probably earning more than $20,000 today plus tips.

The salon owner who was earning approximately $10,000 in 1979 is probably earning around $20,000 today. Inflation has caused the price of all services to rapidly increase, and the products that the salon uses are not increasing in the same proportion. Larger salons were experiencing even more rapid growth during the past three years. More prestigious salons can afford to pay their operators a smaller salary in many cases because the operator wants to benefit by working next to recognized and highly skilled hairstylists. So, you can see that salaries do not always meet with expectations. Ultimately, you will have to choose between accepting a higher salary now, and perhaps having it remain the same for several years, or taking the lesser salary now, with an eye to the future when you have acquired a fine technique.

The franchise owner's salary was projected to be somewhere between $18,000 and $23,000 a year in the 1980s. You can see that the franchise owner's income is similar to the skilled stylist's annual salary.

WORKING CONDITIONS

There may or may not be added benefits for an operator who is employed by a salon. Sometimes group health and life insurance policies cover the operator, and vacations may or may not be included. Paid vacations are now quite common.

The long hours and the pressures of the job should be taken

into consideration. Most of your work will be on the weekends when your patrons want to look their best. Some salons even have Sunday hours. So find out the schedules of the salon where you are contemplating employment and weigh all of the pros and cons carefully. Cosmetology can bring you many hours of pleasure and a wonderfully secure future. The ideal is simply to work at the location and for the number of hours that will make you the happiest.

CHAPTER 17

STATE COSMETOLOGY BOARDS

In every state there is a body that makes the rules and regulations for all cosmetologists, their businesses, and their associations. In California it is called the State Board of Cosmetology, and variations of that title are used in every state. These boards exist to protect you and the public. They can deny your license renewal through revocation or suspension. They can actually enforce disqualification if just cause is shown. So find out about your state's regulations. Be informed.

The state boards were established to protect the consumer, to elevate cosmetology to a higher level, and to maintain that level through the continuation of the board itself.

New members of the board are selected by appointment and hold their given posts for varying numbers of years, depending on the state. In Washington, D.C., there are only three members on the board. The stipulations are that each shall be twenty-five years of age, have practiced cosmetology for five years, be United States citizens, and residents of Washington, D.C. Board members cannot be affiliated with any school of cosmetology while serving on the board.

The members of this particular board must elect a president and a treasurer from the board. Two members constitute a quorum. The board meets at least four times a year.

In North Carolina, a three-member board is appointed by the governor. The board is known as the State Board of Cosmetic

Art Examiners. This board appoints necessary inspectors who are experienced in all areas of cosmetic art. These inspectors make expert reports to the board. Official business of the board includes four annual meetings, supervising and administering examinations, investigations, or inspections. The board also submits a fiscal budget to cover the board's expenses.

In Texas, the Texas Cosmetology Commission consists of six members appointed by the governor. The commission must meet at least once a year. The commission may issue rules, prescribe school curricula for the cosmetology schools, prescribe the content of the examinations, and establish the sanitary rules that pertain to cosmetology.

The Florida State Board of Cosmetology has seven members appointed by the governor. The members of the board are each directly accountable to the governor.

In New York state, the advisory committee is the equivalent of the cosmetology board in other states. This committee consists of five members. It is their job to advise the secretary of state on all matters relating to hairdressing and cosmetology.

California has a seven-member board that administers examinations of all applicants for registration, issues certificates of registration, registers cosmetological establishments and cosmetology schools, reports all violations to proper authorities, holds investigations and inquiries, adopts sanitary rules and regulations, and makes an annual report to the governor concerning the condition of cosmetology and its affiliated branches. A financial statement accompanies this report and lists the expenditures and monies received from fees, licenses, registrations, and applications.

It is important to know the duties performed by your state's board and to know what laws protect you. The governing bodies that create the cosmetology tests and rules affect what you can and cannot do. You should read the specific rules and regulations for the state in which you will be practicing. The state board is a political branch of cosmetology, and you may be interested in being part of it one day. Take an interest in who is making the rules, and write to the state board if you feel that something is unfair. As a cosmetologist, the board represents you at the state level, and you have a stake in its decision.

APPENDIX A

BIBLIOGRAPHY

STATUTES

An Act, issued by the State Board of Cosmetic Art Examiners, Raleigh, North Carolina, to regulate the practice of cosmetic art in the State of North Carolina, 1974.

The Cosmetology Act, including amendments effective on or before January 1, 1980, also excerpts from General Provisions of the Business and Professional Code and the Government Code, issued by Board of Cosmetology, Sacramento, California.

Cosmetology Practice Act, 1981, Government of the District of Columbia, Department of Licenses, Investigations, and Inspections; Board of Cosmetology, 614 H Street, N.W., Washington, D.C.

The Cosmetology Statutes (codified Article 8451A) and its companion, *General Rules and Regulations* including the *Cosmetology Commission Sanitary Rulings,* Texas Cosmetology Commission, Austin, Texas.

Curriculum and Rules for Recognized Schools and Colleges of Beauty Culture, North Carolina State Board of Cosmetic Art Examiners, Raleigh, North Carolina, 1980.

Department of Professional Regulation, 1980, Board of Cosmetology, the Oakland Building, 2009 Apalachee Parkway, Tallahassee, Florida.

Florida License Analysis, Florida State Board of Cosmetology (last amended 1978), Tallahassee, Florida.

Hairdressing and Cosmetology, Statutory Provisions, Rules and Regulations, State Sanitary Code, New York City Health Code, Glossary of Terms, Sample Test Questions, Department of State, Division of Licensing Service, Albany, New York.

Rules and Regulations of the State Board of Cosmetology, includes amendments through March 1981, issued by Board of Cosmetology, Sacramento, California.

SUGGESTED READINGS

Books

Ahearn, Jerry J. *West's Textbook of Cosmetology.* New York: West Publishing Company, 1981.

Cassiday, Doris and Bruce Cassiday. *Careers in the Beauty Industry.* Watts, California: Career Concise Guides Series, 1978.

Colletti, Anthony B. *Revista a los Exámenes de Cosmetología que Hace la Junta Estatal.* Keystone Publications, 1976.

_____. *State Board Review Examinations in Cosmetology.* Keystone Publications, 1976.

Dalton, John W. *The Professional Cosmetologist.* 3rd ed. St. Paul: West Publishing Company, 1985.

Franco, Silvia, et al. *Cosmetology: A Professional Text.* New York: McGraw-Hill, 1980.

Green, Susan. *Salon Management.* Englewood Cliffs, New Jersey: Prentice-Hall, 1984.

Kibbe, Constance. *Standard Textbook of Cosmetology.* New York: Milady Publishing, 1985.

MacDonald, Susan. *Your Career in the Beauty Industry.* New York: Arco Career Guidance Series, 1979.

MacDonald, Susan and Maxine Mottram. *Preparations for Cosmetology Licensing Examinations.* New York: Arco, 1980.

Masters, T.W. *Hairdressing in Theory and Practice.* 6th ed. Hampshire, England: Gower Ltd., 1984.

Milady Publishing Corporation Staff. *The Milady State Board Cosmetology Guide.* New York: Milady Publishing, 1985.

_____. *Van Dean Manual Professional Techniques for Cosmetologists.* rev. ed. Milady, 1977.

Naley, Linda. *Looking Forward to a Career: Cosmetology.* 2d ed. Minneapolis: Dillon, 1976.

Powitt, A. H. *Exam Reviews in Hair Structure and Chemistry.* 4th ed. New York: Milady, 1984.

_____. *Hair Structure and Chemistry Simplified.* New York: Milady Publishing, 1977.

The Prentice-Hall Textbook of Cosmetology. 2d ed. Englewood Cliffs, New Jersey: Prentice-Hall, 1984.

Rudman, Jack. *Cosmetology.* Syosset, New York: National Learning (Occupational Competency Examination Series).

Tezak, E. J. *Exam Reviews in Beauty Salon Management.* Milady, 1974.

_____. *Successful Salon Management for Cosmetology Students.* Milady, 1974.

Wall, Florence E. *Aid to State Board Examinations in Cosmetology.* Keystone Publications, 1975.

Articles

Saturn, P. R. "Barber Shop Haircuts." *Glamour* 82 (December 1984): 80.

Zahn, D. "Hairdressing Olympics: World Championships of Hairdressing." *People Weekly* 22 (September 24, 1984): 129-31.

References

Chiranky, Gary, ed. *Cosmetology Dictionary.* Keystone Publications, 1980.

Colletti, Anthony B. *A Dictionary of Cosmetology and Related Sciences.* Keystone Publications, 1981.

Periodicals

American Hairdresser Salon Owner. Official professional publication of NHCA. New York.

American Hairdresser Salon Owner. Service Publications, Inc., Dayton, Ohio.

International Beauty Show Program (1981). Conventions and Exhibitions, New York.

National Journal of Esthetics. El Segundo, California.

STANDARDS FOR ACCREDITATION

Accreditation means that a school has met national standards of educational performance which have been established by an impartial nongovernmental agency. Cosmetology schools must meet and maintain the following standards, established by the National Accrediting Commission of Cosmetology Arts and Sciences, in order to be accredited.

The school of cosmetology arts and sciences has well-organized curriculums designed to prepare graduates for licensing examinations and for profitable employment.

The ownership and control of the school are publicly stated. Modern methods of organization and administration are employed, and the school is operated on an ethical basis.

Student recruitment reflects sound ethical and legal practices. The school recruits and admits students who have aptitude, interest and motivation to learn and be employable in the field of cosmetology arts and sciences.

Student tuition, fees and refund policies are clearly outlined and completely stated in printed form, and are uniformly administered. Student financial records are maintained, and are current.

The school maintains a supervised and adequately equipped clinic which serves exclusively as a laboratory in which students improve their knowledge and skills in cosmetology science.

The school has a faculty of adequate size qualified by preparation, experience and personality to carry out the objectives of the school.

The school of cosmetology arts and sciences has adequately equipped work stations; secure provisions for storage of equipment, records and supplies; and provides safe working conditions.

The school provides an adequate supply of authoritative and instructional materials and training aids needed in the instruction of each curriculum offered in the overall school program.

Well-developed teaching plans exist for each instructional session, and teaching techniques reflect currently acceptable educational practices.

Each student is given guidance and counseling throughout his or her school career, and assistance in securing employment is provided.

The school is financially sound and able to discharge its responsibilities to its students.

The school is operated as a post-secondary educational institution and maintains the appearance of a school. It must have an officially designated administrative office or center and appropriate classrooms. Areas must be provided for guidance and counseling, library, and other supportive services.

CURRICULUMS AVAILABLE IN ACCREDITED SCHOOLS

A description of some of the curriculum titles used by schools and the general objectives and curriculum descriptions for each code follows.

Advanced Cosmetology

(Schools may use curriculum titles such as: Advanced Cosmetology, Master Cosmetology, Coiffure Creation, Grand Master Hairdresser, Cosmetology II, or Advanced Hairdressing and Cosmetology.)

Objective and curriculum description. The objective of an advanced cosmetology curriculum is to advance the licensed cosmetologist's knowledge and expertise in the industry. Emphasis is placed on improving techniques and perfecting new styles. Instruction is also given on how to improve their financial position in the industry.

Barbering

(Schools may use curriculum titles such as: Barbering, Men's Hairstyling, Barbering/Cosmetology Course, or Barbers Program.)

Objective and curriculum description. The primary objective of the barbering curriculum is to prepare students for the state licensing examination to become a licensed barber. The course of study generally includes cutting and styling, hair coloring, permanent waving, scalp and hair treatments, and shaving. Special emphasis is placed on hair care for men.

Cosmetology

(Schools may use curriculum titles such as: Basic Cosmetology, General Cosmetology, Beauty Culture, Cosmetology, Operator, Hairdressing, Beautician, or Hair Design.)

Objective and curriculum description. The primary objective of the cosmetology curriculum is to prepare students for the state licensing examination to become a licensed cosmetologist. The course of study generally includes cutting and styling, hair coloring, make-up and facials, manicuring and pedicuring, permanent waving, scalp and hair treatments, and other related subjects.

Hair Removal

(Schools may use curriculum titles such as: Hair Removal or Electrolysis.)

Objective and curriculum description. The objective of a hair removal curriculum is to advance the student's knowledge and expertise in the permanent removal of hair. The course of study generally includes machine operation, sanitation and sterilization, posture and positioning, advertisement, salon setups and ethics.

Hair Weaving

Objective and curriculum description. The objective of the hair weaving curriculum is to advance the student's knowledge and expertise in hair weaving and braiding techniques. Emphasis is placed on current styles and creation of new designs.

Manicuring

(Schools may use curriculum titles such as: Manicuring, Cosmetology-Manicurist, Manicurist-Pedicurist, or Manicuring and Sculptured Nails.)

Objective and curriculum description. The objective of the manicuring curriculum is to train the student in nail structures and manicuring techniques. Advanced training may be given in the areas of sculptured nails (application and maintenance), nail wrapping, application of ready-to-wear nails and pedicuring techniques. Some states have a separate licensing examination for manicurists.

Refresher Training

(Schools may use curriculum titles such as: Refresher Training, Brush-up, or Refresher Beauticians.)

Objective and curriculum description. These curriculums are quite varied and are generally designed to meet the individual needs of individuals for brush-up or refresher training in specific areas of cosmetology to prepare them to take the state examination, obtain a position in the field, or improve specific skills.

Salon Management

(Schools may use curriculum titles such as: Manager, Cosmetology Manager, Junior Manager, Salon Management,

Manager Training, Beauty Culture Manager, Operator-Manager, Beauty Salon Manager, Master Salon Management or Beauty Culture Manager.)

Objective and curriculum description. This curriculum is designed to prepare graduate cosmetologists to assume salon management positions or to successfully open their own salons. Emphasis is placed in the areas of good business techniques and practices, common management problems and issues, potential salon problems and their correction and prevention. Some states offer a separate license for salon managers.

Shampoo Specialist

(Schools may use curriculum titles such as: Shampoo Specialist, Shampoo and Conditioning Specialist, Shampoo Technician, or Shampoo Assistant.)

Objective and curriculum description. The purpose of the shampoo specialist curriculum is to train the student in proper shampooing techniques and conditioning of the hair. Emphasis is placed on scalp and skin disorders and product knowledge.

Skin Care

(Schools may use curriculum titles such as: Aesthetician, Cosmetician, Esthetics, Facialist, Make-Up, Master Skin Care and Professional Make-Up, or Salon Make-Up.)

Objective and curriculum decription. The objective of the skin care curriculum is to advance the student's knowledge in the specialized area of skin care and make-up. Special emphasis is placed on diagnosis and treatment of various skin disorders/conditions, professional approach to make-up application, and facial techniques.

Teacher Training

(Schools may use curriculum titles such as: Instructor Training, Junior Instructor, Teacher Trainee, Master Teacher, Student Instructor, Instructor Course, Beauty Culture Teacher, Cadet Teacher, or Theory Instructor.)

Objective and curriculum description. The teacher training curriculum is designed to prepare the licensed cosmetologist to become a licensed instructor. Instruction in public speaking, audiovisual aids, state board examination, teaching methods, lesson planning, and testing/grading is emphasized.

Unisex

Objective and curriculum description. The purpose of this curriculum is to train the student in the techniques of both men's and women's hair care.

Wig Specialist

(Schools may use curriculum titles such as: Wig Specialist, Wigs, Wiggery, or Wigology.)

Objective and curriculum description. The objective of the wig specialist curriculum is to advance the student's knowledge and expertise in working with wigs and hairpieces. Special emphasis is placed on marketing techniques with the industry, styling, and maintenance of wigs.

Make-Up Specialist

(Schools may use curriculum titles such as: Cosmetician, Make-Up Specialist.)

Objective and curriculum description. The principal objective in the make-up specialist curriculum is knowing how to apply make-up techniques in the correct and most flattering fashion for each patron. The course usually includes the study of various professional cosmetics, the implements, the principles, and the techniques of make-up application.

Sculptured Nails

(Schools may use curriculum titles such as: Sculptured Nails, Nail Design, Artificial Nails, Advanced Nails.)

Objective and curriculum description. The curriculum generally is designed to train students in advanced nail care, such as nail repair, oil manicures, nail building, and nail wrapping.

Hair Coloring

(Schools may use curriculum titles such as: Hair Coloring, Hair Dying, Permanent Coloring, Hair Tinting, Frosting, Bleaching.)

Objective and curriculum description. The hair coloring curriculum is designed to train the student in the proper techniques used for applying temporary or permanent colors, as well as the steps in lightening or toning a patron's hair.

Hair Cutting

(Schools may use curriculum titles such as: Hair Cutting, Hair Shaping, Advanced Cutting.)

Objective and curriculum description. The primary objective in the hair cutting curriculum is to train students to use the proper implements with the proper technique to give the patron the hairstyle (cut) requested.

Permanent Waving

(Schools may use curriculum titles such as: Body Waving, Cold Waving, Chemical Waving.)

Objective and curriculum description. The permanent waving curriculum is designed to advance the student's knowledge and expertise in the techniques for curling hair. The primary objective is to train students in using professional cold waving chemicals and implements.

Black Hair Studies

(Schools may use curriculum titles such as: Chemical Relaxing, Hair Straightening, Hair Silking, Hair Pressing.)

Objective and curriculum description. The objective of the black hair studies is to prepare the student in curl reduction or straightening. Emphasis is usually placed on hair relaxing to permit greater manageability of the hair.

STATE BOARDS OF COSMETOLOGY

Most states (including the District of Columbia and Puerto Rico) have a state cosmetology board which sets requirements for schools, salons, and individual cosmetologists. The rules vary from state to state. For example, the number of hours of training required varies from 1000 hours (New York, Massachusetts, Oklahoma, Puerto Rico) to 2500 hours (Oregon). Almost half (23 states) require 1500 hours. If you want to know the rules for a particular state you should write directly to the state board for this information. The address and telephone number of the state boards is listed below.

ALABAMA BOARD OF COSMETOLOGY
  First Southern Federal Tower
  100 Commerce Street, Suite 801
  Montgomery, Alabama 36130
  (205) 832-5074

ALASKA BOARD OF BARBERS
AND HAIRDRESSERS
  Department of Commerce
    and Economic Development
  Division of Occupational
    Licensing
  Pouch D
  Juneau, Alaska 99811
  (907) 465-2547

ARIZONA STATE BOARD
OF COSMETOLOGY
  1625 W. Jefferson, Room 125
  Phoenix, Arizona 85007
  (602) 255-5301

ARKANSAS STATE BOARD OF COSMETOLOGY
  1515 West Seventh Street
  Suite 400
  Little Rock, Arkansas 72202
  (501) 371-2168

CALIFORNIA STATE BOARD
OF COSMETOLOGY
  Department of Consumer Affairs
  1020 N. Street
  Sacramento, California 95814
  (916) 445-5863

COLORADO BOARD OF BARBERS
AND COSMETOLOGISTS
  1525 Sherman Street, Room 606
  Denver, Colorado 80203
  (303) 866-2501

CONNECTICUT STATE DEPARTMENT OF
HEALTH SERVICES
  Division of Medical Quality Assurance
  150 Washington Street
  Hartford, Connecticut 06115
  (203) 566-4068

DELAWARE BOARD OF
PERSONAL SERVICES
  Margaret O'Neill Building
  2nd Floor
  P.O. Box 1401
  Dover, Delaware 19903
  (302) 736-4796

DISTRICT OF COLUMBIA
BOARD OF COSMETOLOGY
  614 H Street, N.W., Room 923
  Washington, DC 20001
  (202) 727-6215

FLORIDA STATE BOARD OF
COSMETOLOGY
130 North Monroe Street
Suite 15
Tallahassee, Florida 32301
(904) 488-5702

GEORGIA STATE BOARD OF
COSMETOLOGY
166 Pryor Street, S.W.
Atlanta, Georgia 30303
(404) 656-3909

HAWAII BOARD OF COSMETOLOGY
Professional and Vocational
Licensing Division
Department of Commerce
and Consumer Affairs
P.O. Box 3469
Honolulu, Hawaii 96801
(808) 548-7461

IDAHO STATE BOARD OF
COSMETOLOGY
2404 Bank Drive
Room 312
Boise, Idaho 83705
(208) 334-3233

ILLINOIS DEPARTMENT OF
REGISTRATION AND EDUCATION
Beauty Culture Section
320 West Washington Street
3rd Floor
Springfield, Illinois 62786
(217) 785-0800

INDIANA BOARD OF BEAUTY
CULTURIST EXAMINERS
1021 State Office Building
100 N. Senate Avenue
Indianapolis, Indiana 46204
(317) 232-3932

IOWA COSMETOLOGY
BOARD OF EXAMINERS
  Lucas State Office Building
  Des Moines, Iowa 50319
  (515) 281-4422

KANSAS STATE BOARD OF
COSMETOLOGY
  630 Kansas Avenue
  Topeka, Kansas 66603
  (913) 296-3155

KENTUCKY STATE BOARD
OF HAIRDRESSERS AND
COSMETOLOGISTS
  314 W. Second Street
  Frankfort, Kentucky 40601
  (502) 827-4951

LOUISIANA STATE BOARD
OF COSMETOLOGY
  Colonial Bank Building
  2714 Canal Street, Room 412
  New Orleans, Louisiana 70119
  (504) 568-5267

MAINE STATE BOARD
OF COSMETOLOGY
  Capitol Shopping Center
  Western Avenue
  State House Station 62
  Augusta, Maine 04333
  (207) 289-2231

MARYLAND STATE BOARD
OF COSMETOLOGISTS
  501 St. Paul Place, Room 803
  Baltimore, Maryland 21202
  (301) 659-6320

MASSACHUSETTS BOARD OF
REGISTRATION OF HAIRDRESSERS
  Leverett Saltonstall Building
  100 Cambridge Street
  Boston, Massachusetts 02202
  (617) 727-3090

MICHIGAN STATE BOARD
OF COSMETOLOGY
  905 Southland
  P.O. Box 30018
  Lansing, Michigan 48909
  (517) 373-0580

MINNESOTA DEPARTMENT OF
COMMERCE, COSMETOLOGY UNIT
  Metro Square Building
  7th and Roberts Streets
  St. Paul, Minnesota 55101
  (612) 296-8456

MISSISSIPPI STATE BOARD
OF COSMETOLOGY
  1804 North State Street
  Jackson, Mississippi 39202
  (601) 354-6623

MISSOURI STATE BOARD
OF COSMETOLOGY
  3523 N. Ten Mile Drive
  P.O. Box 1062
  Jefferson City, Missouri 65101
  (314) 751-2334

MONTANA STATE BOARD
OF COSMETOLOGISTS
  1424 9th Avenue
  Helena, Montana 59620
  (406) 449-3737

NEBRASKA STATE BOARD OF
COSMETOLOGIST EXAMINERS
  Nebraska State Department of
    Health, Bureau of Examining
    Boards
  301 Centennial Mall South
  P.O. Box 95007
  Lincoln, Nebraska 68509
  (402) 471-2115

NEVADA STATE BOARD
OF COSMETOLOGISTS
   1785 E. Sahara Avenue
   Suite 470
   Las Vegas, Nevada 89109
   (702) 386-5231

NEW HAMPSHIRE BOARD
OF COSMETOLOGY
   Health & Welfare Building
   Hazen Drive
   Concord, New Hampshire 03301
   (603) 271-3608

NEW JERSEY BOARD OF
BEAUTY CULTURE CONTROL
   1100 Raymond Boulevard
   Newark, New Jersey 07102
   (201) 648-2450

NEW MEXICO STATE BOARD
OF COSMETOLOGISTS
   Maya Building, Suite C
   440 Cerrillos Road
   Santa Fe, New Mexico 87501
   (505) 827-7347

NEW YORK DEPARTMENT OF STATE,
DIVISION OF LICENSING SERVICES
   270 Broadway
   New York, New York 10017
   (212) 587-5747

NORTH CAROLINA STATE BOARD
OF COSMETIC ARTS
   P.O. Box 1108
   113 W. Hargett Street
   Raleigh, North Carolina 27602
   (919) 832-1732

NORTH DAKOTA STATE BOARD
OF HAIRDRESSERS
   P.O. Box 1544
   Grand Forks, North Dakota 58201
   (701) 772-1959

OHIO STATE BOARD OF
COSMETOLOGY
 8 East Long Street
 Suite 1000
 Columbus, Ohio 43215
 (614) 466-3834

OKLAHOMA STATE BOARD
OF COSMETOLOGY
 4001 N. Lincoln Boulevard
 Suite 304
 Oklahoma City, Oklahoma 73105
 (405) 521-2441

OREGON BOARD OF BARBERS
AND HAIRDRESSERS
 403 Labor & Industries Building
 Salem, Oregon 97310
 (503) 378-8667

PENNSYLVANIA STATE BOARD
OF COSMETOLOGY
 P.O. Box 2649
 Harrisburg, Pennsylvania 17120
 (717) 787-2478

PUERTO RICO BOARD OF
EXAMINERS OF BEAUTY
SPECIALISTS
 P.O. Box 3271
 San Juan, Puerto Rico 00904
 (809) 725-0142

RHODE ISLAND STATE BOARD
OF HAIRDRESSING
 209 Cannon Building
 75 Davis Street
 Providence, Rhode Island 02908
 (401) 277-2511

SOUTH CAROLINA STATE BOARD
OF COSMETOLOGY
 1209 Blanding Street
 Columbia, South Carolina 29201
 (803) 758-3371

SOUTH DAKOTA COSMETOLOGY
COMMISSION
  AGC Building
  P.O. Box 127
  Pierre, South Dakota 57501
  (605) 224-5072

TENNESSEE STATE BOARD
OF COSMETOLOGY
  706 Church Street
  Suite 516
  Nashville, Tennessee 37219
  (615) 741-2515

TEXAS COSMETOLOGY COMMISSION
  1111 Rio Grande
  Austin, Texas 78701
  (512) 475-3304

UTAH STATE BOARD
OF COSMETOLOGY
  Division of Registration
  160 E. 300 South
  P.O. Box 5802
  Salt Lake City, Utah 84110
  (801) 530-6628

VERMONT STATE BOARD
OF COSMETOLOGY
  Secretary of State's Office
  Division of Licensing and
    Registration
  Pavilion Building
  109 State Street
  Montpelier, Vermont 05602
  (802) 828-2363

VIRGINIA BOARD OF
COSMETOLOGY
  3600 W. Broad Street
  Richmond, Virginia 23230
  (804) 786-8509

WASHINGTON STATE
COSMETOLOGY EXAMINING
COMMITTEE
  P.O. Box 9649
  Olympia, Washington 98504
  (206) 753-3834

WEST VIRGINIA STATE BOARD
OF BARBERS AND BEAUTICIANS
  Gutherie Facilities
  4860 Brenda Lane
  Charleston, West Virginia 25312
  (304) 348-3450

WISCONSIN COSMETOLOGY
EXAMINING BOARD
  P.O. Box 8936
  Madison, Wisconsin 53708
  (608) 266-1630

WYOMING STATE BOARD
OF COSMETOLOGY
  P.O. Box 4480
  Casper, Wyoming 82604
  (307) 265-2917

VGM CAREER BOOKS

OPPORTUNITIES IN

*Available in both
paperback and hardbound
editions*

Accounting Careers
Acting Careers
Advertising Careers
Agriculture Careers
Airline Careers
Animal and Pet Care
Appraising Valuation Science
Architecture
Automotive Service
Banking
Beauty Culture
Biological Sciences
Book Publishing Careers
Broadcasting Careers
Building Construction Trades
Business Communication Careers
Business Management
Cable Television
Carpentry Careers
Chemical Engineering
Chemistry Careers
Child Care Careers
Chiropractic Health Care
Civil Engineering Careers
Commercial Art and Graphic
 Design
Computer Aided Design
 and Computer Aided Mfg.
Computer Maintenance Careers
Computer Science Careers
Counseling & Development
Crafts Careers
Dance
Data Processing Careers
Dental Care
Drafting Careers
Electrical Trades
Electronic and Electrical
 Engineering
Energy Careers
Engineering Technology Careers
Environmental Careers
Fashion Careers
Federal Government Careers
Film Careers
Financial Careers
Fire Protection Services
Fitness Careers
Food Services
Foreign Language Careers
Forestry Careers
Gerontology Careers
Government Service
Graphic Communications

Health and
 Medical Careers
High Tech Careers
Home Economics Careers
Hospital Administration
Hotel & Motel Management
Industrial Design
Insurance Careers
Interior Design
International Business
Journalism Careers
Landscape Architecture
Laser Technology
Law Careers
Law Enforcement and
 Criminal Justice
Library and Information
 Science
Machine Trades
Magazine Publishing Careers
Management
Marine & Maritime Careers
Marketing Careers
Materials Science
Mechanical Engineering
Microelectronics
Modeling Careers
Music Careers
Nursing Careers
Nutrition Careers
Occupational Therapy
 Careers
Office Occupations
Opticianry
Optometry
Packaging Science
Paralegal Careers
Paramedical Careers
Part-time & Summer Jobs
Personnel Management
Pharmacy Careers
Photography
Physical Therapy Careers
Plumbing & Pipe Fitting
Podiatric Medicine
Printing Careers
Psychiatry
Psychology
Public Health Careers
Public Relations Careers
Real Estate
Recreation and Leisure
Refrigeration and
 Air Conditioning
Religious Service
Retailing
Robotics Careers
Sales Careers

Sales & Marketing
Secretarial Careers
Securities Industry
Social Work Careers
Speech-Language Pathology
 Careers
Sports & Athletics
Sports Medicine
State and Local Government
Teaching Careers
Technical Communications
Telecommunications
Television and Video Careers
Theatrical Design
 & Production
Transportation Careers
Travel Careers
Veterinary Medicine Careers
Vocational and Technical Careers
Word Processing
Writing Careers
Your Own Service Business

CAREERS IN
Accounting
Business
Communications
Computers
Health Care
Science

CAREER DIRECTORIES
Careers Encyclopedia
Occupational Outlook Handbook

CAREER PLANNING
How to Get and Get Ahead
 On Your First Job
How to Get People to Do
 Things Your Way
How to Have a Winning
 Job Interview
How to Land a Better Job
How to Write a Winning Résumé
Joyce Lain Kennedy's Career Book
Life Plan
Planning Your Career Change
Planning Your Career of
 Tomorrow
Planning Your College Education
Planning Your Military Career
Planning Your Own Home
 Business
Planning Your Young Child's
 Education

SURVIVAL GUIDES
High School Survival Guide
College Survival Guide

VGM Career Horizons
a division of *NTC Publishing Group*
4255 West Touhy Avenue
Lincolnwood, Illinois 60646-1975

WITHDRAWAL